Building
STRENGTH
AND STAMINA

New Nautilus Training for Total Fitness

Wayne Westcott, PhD
South Shore YMCA, Quincy, MA

Nautilus International

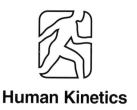

Human Kinetics

Library of Congress Cataloging-in-Publication Data

Westcott, Wayne L., 1949-
  Building strength and stamina : new Nautilus training for total
fitness / Wayne Westcott and Nautilus International.
     p.   cm.
  Includes bibliographical references (p.   ) and index.
  ISBN 0-88011-550-5
  1. Physical fitness. 2. Exercise. 3. Nautilus weight training
equipment.   I. Nautilus International (Firm)   II. Title.
  GV481.W47   1996
  613.7'1--dc20   96-15784
                                                                         CIP

ISBN: 0-88011-550-5

Developmental Editor: Elaine Mustain; **Assistant Editors:** Susan Moore, Jacqueline Blakley, and Sandra Merz Bott; **Editorial Assistant:** Amy Carnes; **Copyeditor:** Bonnie Pettifor; **Proofreader:** Erin Cler; **Indexer:** Diana Witt; **Graphic Designer:** Robert Reuther; **Graphic Artist:** Denise Lowry; **Photo Editor:** Boyd LaFoon; **Cover Designer:** Keith Blomberg; **Photographer (cover):** John Beckett; **Photographers (interior):** John Beckett; **Illustrator:** William Humbart; **Printer:** United Graphics

Note. All interior photographs were taken by John Beckett, with the exceptions of photos by Mary Ann Halpin, p.46; Wayne Westcott, p. 149; CLEO Photography, p. 150; George Monserrat, p. 151; Kerry Loughman, p. 161; and Bruce Bennett Studios, p. 215.

Printed in the United States of America   10 9 8 7 6 5 4 3 2 1

Human Kinetics
Web site: http://www.humankinetics.com/

United States: Human Kinetics, P.O. Box 5076, Champaign, IL 61825-5076
1-800-747-4457
e-mail: humank@hkusa.com

Canada: Human Kinetics, Box 24040, Windsor, ON N8Y 4Y9
1-800-465-7301 (in Canada only)
e-mail: humank@hkcanada.com

Europe: Human Kinetics, P.O. Box IW14, Leeds LS16 6TR, United Kingdom
(44) 1132 781708
e-mail: humank@hkeurope.com

Australia: Human Kinetics, 57A Price Avenue, Lower Mitcham, South Australia 5062
(08) 277 1555
e-mail: humank@hkaustralia.com

New Zealand: Human Kinetics, P.O. Box 105-231, Auckland 1
(09) 523 3462
e-mail: humank@hknewz.com

Contents

Acknowledgments

The author and Nautilus International wish to acknowledge the invaluable assistance of our esteemed colleagues, Bill Rodgers, Bob Sweeney, Candice Copeland Brooks, Douglas Brooks, Ted Miller, Elaine Mustain, Ralph Yohe, Mary Moore, Cyndi Skaar, and Danny Stanton. We especially appreciate the professional contributions of Susan Ramsden who typed the manuscripts; William Humbart who produced the artwork; John Beckett, Joanne Gardner, Jeffrey Goodman, and Herita Jones who produced the photographs; Terry Alexander, Bill Amadio, Heather Dunn, Shannon Godfrey, Ken Green, Julie Horanski, Lee Ann Jefferies, and Jeff Martin who demonstrated the exercises; Rita La Rosa Loud who oversees the South Shore YMCA research classes; Claudia Westcott who directs the South Shore YMCA Nautilus Fitness Center; and God's grace in the design and development of this book.

Introduction

You may know people who take better care of their automobiles than they do of their bodies. Unfortunately, just driving the best-maintained motor vehicle wears it out. Not the human body! Regular exercise helps your body function better and last longer. A well-conditioned 50-year-old may be in better physical shape than a sedentary 20-year-old. This is why your activity and exercise habits have a major impact on your health and fitness.

Your muscles are the engines of your body. Strong muscles enable you to function like an eight-cylinder sports car, while weak muscles provide less power than a motor scooter. If you are out of shape, you may wonder whether it's really possible to develop your underconditioned muscular system. The answer is a resounding "Yes!" Men and women of all ages can increase their overall muscle strength by more than 50 percent with just two months of strength training. A strong muscular system feels and functions better and reduces your risk of many degenerative problems associated with aging. And because your muscles also serve as the chassis of the body, strength training can improve your physical appearance.

A strong heart is just as important to good health as strong skeletal muscles. Of course, the heart is also a muscle that works as the fuel pump of the body transporting fuel and oxygen to the muscles and other tissues. Because heart disease is the leading cause of death in most affluent societies, you should give cardiovascular fitness high priority. Regular endurance exercise improves the pumping capacity of your heart and makes your circulatory system more efficient, benefiting your heart and all body tissues. For example, as your heart becomes stronger it pumps more blood each time it contracts and so beats less frequently. Endurance training may reduce your resting heart rate by 20 beats a minute, which saves almost 30,000 heart beats every day.

But what if you don't have time to spend a couple of hours at the fitness center every day? Good news! *Building Strength and Stamina* will help you implement a personal fitness program that produces more strength and stamina than you probably thought possible. The exercise progressions are safe, and the time commitment is manageable. The recommended strength training program requires about 25 minutes a session, three days a week. This is enough to achieve high levels of muscular fitness. Add a warm-up, a 25-minute endurance training session, and a cool-down to each workout, and one hour a day, three days a week, should help you experience a new quality of life, including more physical activity, lower weight, and better sport performance. A reasonable time investment for a better body and enhanced physical fitness!

Over 90 percent of the thousands of men and women trained to use this simple and successful exercise program have continued to be physically active. The muscle gain, fat loss, new strength, and increased stamina experienced by these previously sedentary adults convinced them that three hours of sensible exercise makes for a much better week.

As you read *Building Strength and Stamina*, keep in mind that it is a book designed for doers. Reading it will make you more knowledgeable, but it will not make you more physically fit. To benefit most from this book, first obtain your physician's permission, then begin the exercise programs at the appropriate level. If you are already doing strength training, add endurance training. If you are already doing endurance training, start strength training. A well-designed and balanced fitness program is hard to beat!

Be sure to exercise sensibly and avoid overtraining, because doing too much too soon can cause injury. And injury can cause you to quit training altogether. Rest days are essential for maximizing your muscular strength and cardiovascular endurance. Follow the training guidelines, progress gradually, and experience firsthand the many benefits of physical fitness.

CHAPTER 1

How Fit Can You Get?

Do you want to exercise regularly? You must—since you're reading this book. Your desire to become more physically fit is shared by only a minority: Less than 10 percent of American adults exercise enough to gain measurable fitness benefits (1).

STRENGTH AND ENDURANCE EXERCISE

If you want to get into shape for better sport performance, keep in mind that athletes often fail to develop well-balanced fitness due to one-dimensional, sport-specific training. Football players stress strength and power exercises but may neglect aerobic conditioning. Distance runners emphasize endurance training but may pay little attention to strength development.

Building Strength and Stamina incorporates a complete training program, combining muscle-strengthening exercises with aerobic activity. By following this training program, you can achieve both better general fitness and superior sport conditioning.

Importance of Strength Exercise

The primary purpose of strength exercise is to improve your muscle function. Resistance exercise will make you feel like the high-performance person you'd like to be. It will also develop stronger bones, tendons, and ligaments, enabling you to achieve more in all physical activities. It also

1

reduces your risk of medical problems, including low back pain, illnesses such as diabetes, and degenerative problems such as osteoporosis.

While it is obvious that fit muscles enhance your personal appearance, strength training has another great advantage you may not be aware of. If you struggle with keeping your weight down, it's the activity for you! Regular strength training not only increases your daily energy expenditure, it also boosts your resting metabolism (2). It enables you to burn more calories all day long and so achieve and maintain a more desirable body weight.

Importance of Endurance Exercise

The primary purpose of endurance exercise is to improve your cardiovascular system. This includes your heart, lungs, and blood vessels, which are similar to the fueling and cooling systems in a car. Some of the more obvious outcomes of cardiovascular conditioning include a lower resting heart rate, reduced resting blood pressure, improved exercise performance, and faster physical recovery after exercise of any kind.

Aerobic fitness and cardiovascular health are closely related. The same aerobic adaptations that produce better endurance performance also reduce your risk of coronary artery disease, stroke, and other cardiovascular illnesses.

When combined with strength exercise, endurance activity enables your muscles to use energy more efficiently. And endurance training effectively burns extra calories, reducing body fat.

REALISTIC EXPECTATIONS

Despite the benefits of strength and endurance training, it's important to understand how inherited physical factors influence your fitness potential. Such knowledge enables you to establish realistic training goals and to follow sensible exercise guidelines. No matter who you are, you can become more fit, but it's important to understand the in-born limits you may have to accept.

Strength Potential

We all have the potential to increase our muscle size and strength within certain limitations. No matter what your gender or age, you can improve your muscular fitness through well-designed strength training programs. You may be surprised to learn, however, that age, gender, bodybuild and muscle fiber type all affect your potential for strength development.

Age
People often believe that boys and girls under 15 years are too young, and men and women 55 years and older are too old, to benefit from strength training. In fact, people of all ages can increase their muscle size and strength through a basic program of resistance exercise.

In one study, over 400 participants performed eight weeks of standard Nautilus exercise (3). All of the program participants significantly increased their lean (muscle) weight. The youths (average age of 12 years) added 4.0 pounds of lean weight, the younger adults (average age of 45 years) added 3.0 pounds of lean weight, and the seniors (average age of 65 years) added 3.0 pounds of lean weight (see figure 1.1).

Of course, part of the youth gain in lean weight was due to normal growth processes. But notice that the seniors increased their muscle mass as much as the younger adults. These results are similar to other studies on senior strength exercise and indicate that seniors can build muscle tissue at the same rate as younger adults (4-5).

Likewise, both the senior and younger adult participants increased their strength performance by 50-60 percent over the eight-week training period. The youth participants showed a higher rate of strength performance (60-75 percent over the same training duration), which, as in the case of lean weight gain, was most likely due to normal maturation processes (6-7).

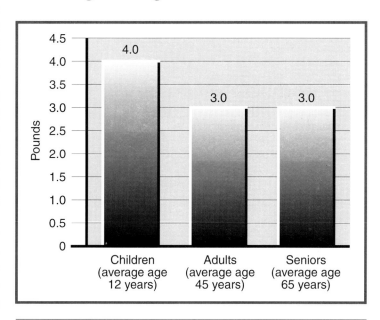

Fig. 1.1 Muscle gains after two months of strength training in three age groups (431 subjects).

Some people may question the advisability of regular resistance exercise for youth and seniors. But properly performed strength training is a safe and productive form of exercise for people of all ages. All of the youth, younger adult, and senior participants in this study remained injury-free throughout the course of the eight-week program.

Gender

Obviously, the average man is larger and stronger than the average woman. Males do have more muscle mass than females. This fact has led many people to believe that women are inherently weak and so can benefit little from a program of strength exercise. When analyzed on a pound-for-pound basis, however, men and women are quite similar in their strength capacity.

A large research study assessed quadriceps strength in 907 trained men and women (8). As illustrated in table 1.1, the men completed 10 leg extensions with 119 pounds, and the women completed 10 leg extensions with 79 pounds. But when researchers compared men and women on the basis of body weight, the men performed 10 repetitions with 62 percent of their body weight, and the women performed 10 repetitions with 55 percent of their body weight.

Table 1.1

Quadriceps strength for men and women as measured by the 10-repetition maximum weight load on the Nautilus leg extension machine (907 subjects).

	Men	Women
Age (in years)	43	42
Body weight (in pounds)	191	143
10-repetition maximum (pounds)	119	79
Strength quotient (body weight)	62%	55%
Strength quotient (lean body weight)	74%	73%

Although assessing quadriceps strength on the basis of body weight narrows the gender gap, it still does not compare strength fairly between men and women. This is because men have less fat weight and more lean weight than women. Therefore, the researchers also compared performance based on the subjects' estimated lean weight. This comparison showed that both the men and women performed 10 leg extensions with a weight load equal to about 75 percent of their lean weight. So men and women have similar levels of quadriceps strength when evaluated on a lean weight basis.

Other studies involving hundreds of men and women have shown similar gains in muscle size and strength for both genders after several weeks of resistance training (3). It is clear that men and women have comparable lean weight strength and that they can benefit equally from sensible strength training.

As you can see, no matter your age or gender, you can achieve significant increases in both your muscle size and strength through properly performed strength training.

Bodybuild

Generally speaking, there are four basic body types (see figure 1.2). A linear appearance characterizes the ectomorphic physique. Ectomorphs have relatively low amounts of muscle and fat. They are typically light in body weight and are best suited for endurance activities such as distance running.

The mesomorphic physique is rectangular in appearance. Mesomorphs have relatively high amounts of muscle and relatively low amounts of fat. They are typically medium in body weight and are best suited for strength activities such as wrestling and gymnastics.

The endomorphic physique looks more rounded than the others. Endomorphs have relatively low amounts of muscle, but relatively high amounts of fat. A variation is the endomesomorph, who has relatively high amounts of both muscle and fat. Endomesomorphs are typically heavy for their heights and are best suited for power activities, such as football, in which large size is an advantage.

Although mesomorphs have the greatest potential to develop muscular physiques, ectomorphs and endomorphs can also add significant amounts of muscle through sensible strength training. Ectomorphs typically achieve more muscular physiques when they increase their daily consumption of nutritious foods, with attention to sufficient protein and complex carbohy-

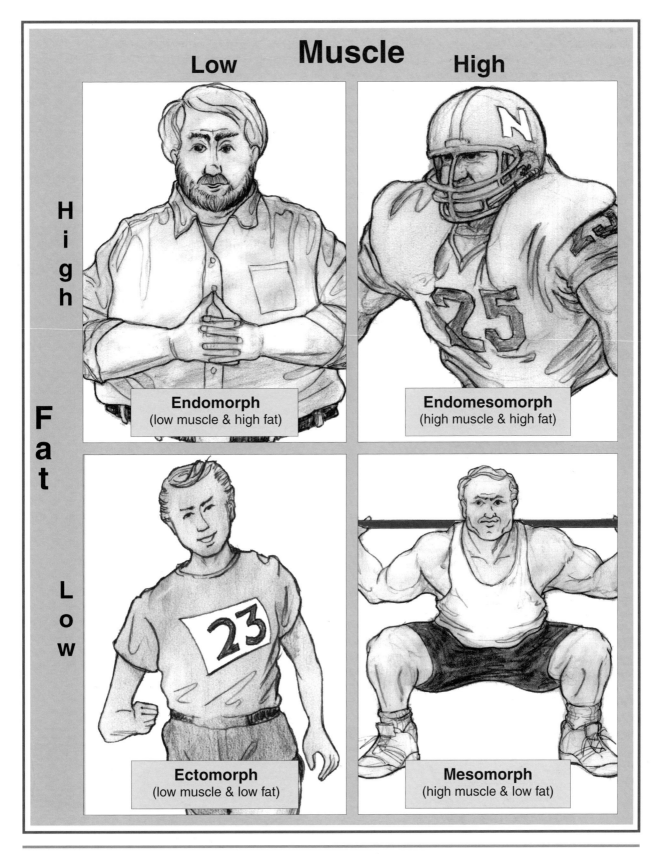

Fig. 1.2 Relative amounts of muscle and fat for endomorphic, endomesomorphic, ectomorphic, and mesomorphic individuals.

drates. Endomorphs and endomesomorphs may benefit from a nutrition program that emphasizes a low-fat, moderate-calorie diet.

Limb Length

Strength performance has a lot to do with the lever systems formed by our muscles, tendons, and bones. Other things being equal, people with shorter levers (arms and legs) have a strength advantage over people with longer levers. The formula for determining how much resistance your biceps can hold at a right angle is

$$\frac{\text{Muscle force} \times \text{Muscle lever}}{\text{Resistance lever}} = \text{Resistance}$$

Let's assume that your biceps produces 300 pounds of force and that you have a one-inch muscle lever (distance from your elbow joint to your muscle insertion point, which will be discussed further below). If you have a 10-inch resistance lever (forearm), you can hold a 30-pound dumbbell at a right angle (see figure 1.3a). But if you have a 12-inch resistance lever (forearm), you can hold only a 25-pound dumbbell at a right angle (see figure 1.3b). Although the muscle force and muscle insertion points are the same, the shorter forearm provides a distinct strength advantage.

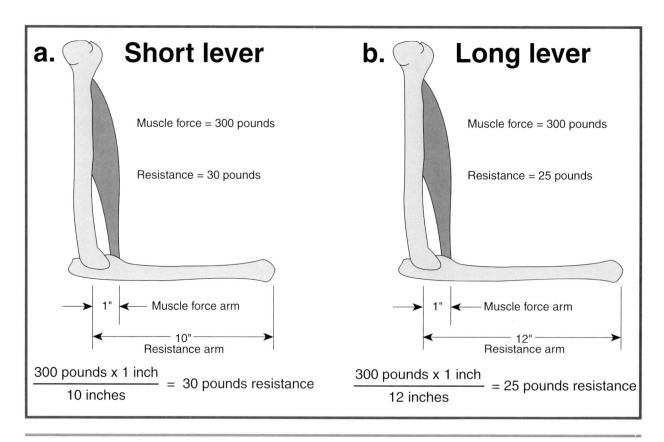

Fig. 1.3 Shorter limb length provides a leverage advantage over longer limb length.

Muscle Insertion Point

Another leverage factor that has a major influence on strength performance is your muscle insertion point. This is the distance between your joint and your muscle attachment that functions as the muscle lever. Generally, people who have muscle insertion points that are farther from the joint have a strength advantage over persons with closer muscle insertion points. Once again, the formula for determining how much resistance your biceps can hold at a right angle is

$$\frac{\text{Muscle force} \times \text{Muscle lever}}{\text{Resistance lever}} = \text{Resistance}$$

Let's again assume that your biceps produces 300 pounds of force, and that your forearm forms a 10-inch resistance lever. If you have a 1.2-inch muscle lever (distance from your elbow to your muscle insertion point), you can hold a 36-pound dumbbell at a right angle (see figure 1.4a). But if you have a 1.0-inch muscle lever, you can hold only a 30-pound dumbbell at a right angle (see figure 1.4b). Although the muscle force and forearm length are the same, the farther tendon insertion point provides a definite strength advantage.

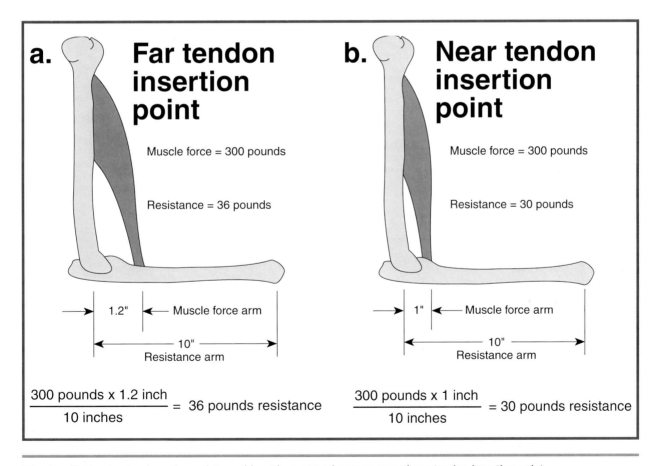

a. **Far tendon insertion point**

Muscle force = 300 pounds

Resistance = 36 pounds

1.2" ← Muscle force arm

10"
Resistance arm

$$\frac{\text{300 pounds x 1.2 inch}}{\text{10 inches}} = 36 \text{ pounds resistance}$$

b. **Near tendon insertion point**

Muscle force = 300 pounds

Resistance = 30 pounds

1" ← Muscle force arm

10"
Resistance arm

$$\frac{\text{300 pounds x 1 inch}}{\text{10 inches}} = 30 \text{ pounds resistance}$$

Fig. 1.4 Farther tendon insertion point provides a leverage advantage over closer tendon insertion point.

Muscle Length

When you compare the length of a muscle with its connecting tendon, you will find different people have different ratios of muscle length to tendon length. Most people have medium-length muscles with medium-length tendons, while some people have relatively short muscles with long tendons, and others have relatively long muscles with short tendons (see figure 1.5).

People who have relatively short muscles have a lower potential for building large muscle size, while those with relatively long muscles have a higher potential for building large muscle size. Although everyone has the capacity to build larger muscles, most successful bodybuilders have the genetic advantage of relatively long muscles throughout their bodies.

To estimate the relative length of your biceps, make a hard biceps contraction with your elbow at a right angle and your wrist turned inward. Now, place as many fingers as possible between your forearm and the end of the bulge your biceps makes. If you can place three fingers in the gap you have relatively short biceps. If you can place two fingers in the gap you have medium length biceps, and if you can place only one finger in the gap you have relatively long biceps.

Muscle Fiber Type

Our muscles are composed of two basic types of contracting cells, known as slow-twitch fibers (type I) and fast-twitch fibers (type II). Slow-twitch

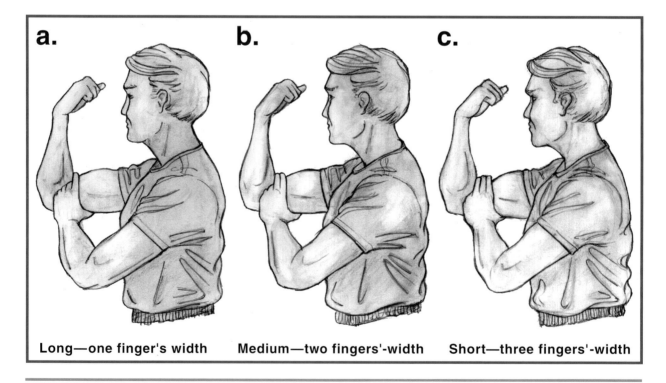

a. **b.** **c.**

Long—one finger's width   Medium—two fingers'-width   Short—three fingers'-width

Fig. 1.5 Estimating relative length of your biceps.

muscle fibers are typically smaller and produce lower levels of force for longer periods of time. Fast-twitch muscle fibers are typically larger and produce higher levels of force for shorter periods of time. While some of our muscles have a majority of slow-twitch fibers, and others have a majority of fast-twitch fibers, most muscles have about the same number of slow-twitch and fast-twitch fibers.

People who inherit a higher than average percentage of slow-twitch fibers generally experience more success in endurance activities, such as distance running. People who inherit a higher than average percentage of fast-twitch fibers are generally more successful in strength activities, such as weightlifting.

Endurance Potential

As with strength conditioning, everyone has the potential to improve cardiovascular endurance. In addition to age, gender, bodybuild, and muscle fiber type, our cardiovascular endurance is related to the ventilation capacity of our lungs, the pumping capacity of our heart, the distribution capacity of our blood vessels, and our blood volume. All of these factors work together to supply our tissues with oxygen. The amount of oxygen we need for basic life processes is relatively small, but vigorous physical activity greatly increases the oxygen needs of our muscles.

Heart and Lung Capacity

When endurance athletes perform high-level aerobic exercise, their lungs may move over 150 liters of air a minute, and their hearts may pump up to 40 liters of blood a minute (9-10). Relative to their body size, endurance athletes have larger lungs, hearts, and arteries than average individuals. They also have more blood vessels and greater blood volume than untrained people. Although endurance training can increase the oxygen utilization capacity of our muscles, its effect on the size of our heart and blood vessels is not fully understood (11). Most likely, successful endurance athletes are genetically endowed with exceptionally effective cardiovascular systems, as well as with favorable muscle physiology.

Age

During our growth years, normal development increases the capacity of our cardiovascular system. But once we reach adulthood, our cardiovascular endurance gradually declines. One reason for this decline is that our maximum heart rate steadily decreases as we age and this reduces the pumping capacity of our heart. As a rule, our maximum heart rate loses about 10 beats a minute every decade. Even so, it is possible for those who haven't been exercising to begin improving their cardiovascular fitness at any age and for those who do exercise regularly to maintain high levels of aerobic endurance throughout their midlife years (12).

Gender

Men typically perform better than women in endurance activities, such as distance running, cycling, and triathlons. This performance advantage is probably due to body composition differences between men and women. Male athletes have a higher percentage of lean weight and a lower percentage of fat weight than female athletes.

Men probably do not have inherently superior cardiovascular systems compared to women. Endurance exercise seems to produce the same physiological adaptations in men and women, and both benefit from regular aerobic activity.

Bodybuild and Composition

Lower body weight is clearly an advantage for endurance activities. This is one reason that almost all successful marathon runners have ectomorphic physiques.

Closely related to bodybuild is body composition. This is the ratio of our fat weight to our lean weight and is expressed as our percent body fat. At a given body weight, people with a lower percent of fat weight and a higher percent of lean weight have an advantage in endurance performance. So one way to increase your aerobic ability is to achieve a lower percentage of body fat through strength training and proper diet.

Muscle Fiber Types

The oxygen receiving capacity of our muscles has as much of an impact on our endurance potential as our cardiovascular, or delivery, system does. Slow-twitch muscle fibers use oxygen more efficiently and so resist fatigue better than fast-twitch fibers. Slow-twitch muscle fibers are best suited to endurance exercise, while fast-twitch muscle fibers are best suited to short duration strength exercise.

SUMMARY

Strength exercise improves our muscular fitness. A strong musculoskeletal system increases our physical performance, reduces our risk of injury, and enhances our personal appearance. Certain genetic characteristics, however, influence our strength potential.

Fortunately, men and women of all ages can improve their muscle strength through a progressive program of resistance exercise. Even if you do not make a major change in your bodybuild as a result of strength training, you will still reap major fitness benefits from it. Stronger muscles, bones, tendons, and ligaments increase your ability to perform physical activity and decrease your risk of musculoskeletal injuries and degenerative diseases. Youth, younger adults, and seniors all benefit from systematic strength exercise. This is good news, because muscle strength is a key factor for overall health and fitness.

Likewise, aerobic exercise improves our cardiovascular fitness. An efficient cardiovascular system benefits both physical performance and health. Even though factors such as basic bodybuild and muscle fiber type have an influence on our endurance potential, men and women of all ages can enhance their cardiovascular endurance through a regular program of aerobic activity.

People who are overweight generally avoid aerobic activities because they find less satisfaction and success in endurance exercise than strength training. But overweight and heavily muscled people should keep in mind that endurance exercise is an excellent way to burn extra calories. Endurance exercise also provides extra protection against heart disease.

Just as a well-maintained engine and fuel system keep a high-performance automobile running well, tuned-up muscular and cardiovascular systems will improve your physical strength and endurance. A combination of strength and endurance fitness will increase your energy level, make you feel and look better, and help you stay healthy longer—all of which will enhance your quality of life. The remaining chapters of this book will help you design effective and efficient strength and endurance exercise programs, enabling you to develop high levels of muscular and cardiovascular fitness.

CHAPTER 2

Fitness and Muscle Strength

So properly performed strength training will make you feel and function better (1). But what specific benefits can you expect from a sensible strength training program? How does your body change in response to resistance exercises to produce these results? And what types of strength training exercises are beneficial?

BENEFITS OF STRENGTH EXERCISE

The primary effect of strength training is to increase both the strength and the size of your muscles. The major muscle groups affected are identified in figure 2.1. But strength training also benefits your bones, tendons, ligaments, and cardiovascular system. Regular strength training reduces your risk of various injuries and illnesses. In addition to the obvious benefits of increased muscle strength, muscle mass, and cardiovascular and muscle endurance, consider the following well-documented but lesser-known reasons why you should make sensible strength exercise a key part of your lifestyle.

Joint Flexibility

You may have heard that strength exercise decreases joint flexibility, but the facts show just the opposite. Research conducted on youth showed that the strength-trained subjects improved their range of joint movement more than the control subjects (2). In a recent study, 48 adult

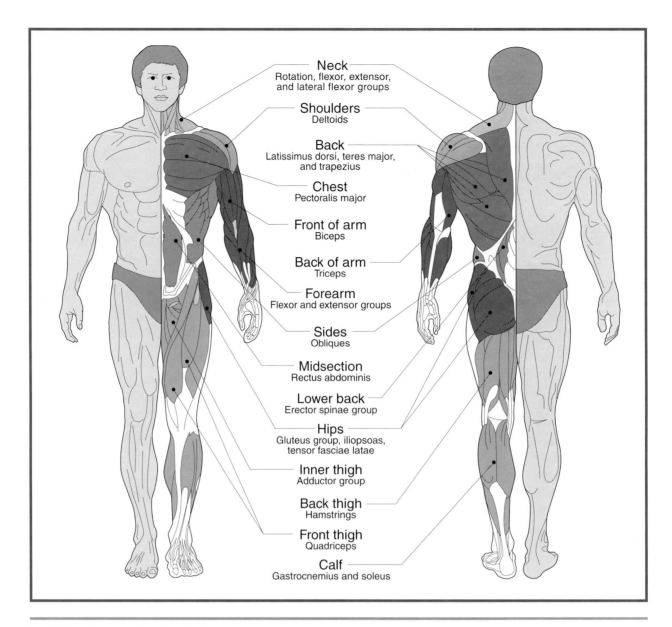

Fig. 2.1 Major muscles of the body.

participants in an eight-week program of Nautilus strength training improved their hip-trunk flexibility by two and one-half inches without performing any stretching exercises. At the same time, they increased their overall muscle strength by 50 percent (3).

These findings indicate that properly performed strength exercise enhances both muscle strength and joint flexibility. High levels of muscle strength and joint flexibility are compatible and can both be attained from full-range strength training.

Body Composition

Body composition refers to the relative amounts of fat tissue and lean tissue in our bodies and is usually expressed as percent body fat. For example, a 100-pound woman who is 25 percent body fat has 25 pounds of fat weight and 75 pounds of lean weight. Generally speaking, males should be less than 15 percent body fat and females should be less than 25 percent body fat.

Adults typically lose five pounds of lean (muscle) weight, and gain 15 pounds of fat weight every decade of life (see figure 2.2). This appears as a 10-pound weight gain on the bathroom scale, but really represents a 20-pound change in our body components. The combined muscle loss and fat gain leads to large increases in our percentage of body fat, which is both unattractive and unhealthy.

If we diet we can reduce our fat weight by consuming fewer calories than we use. Endurance exercise, such as running, cycling, stepping and skating, can also reduce our fat weight by using more calories than we consume. But neither dieting nor endurance exercise replaces our lost muscle tissue.

Muscle gain depends on regular strength exercise, so sensible strength training can improve your body composition. Combine strength training

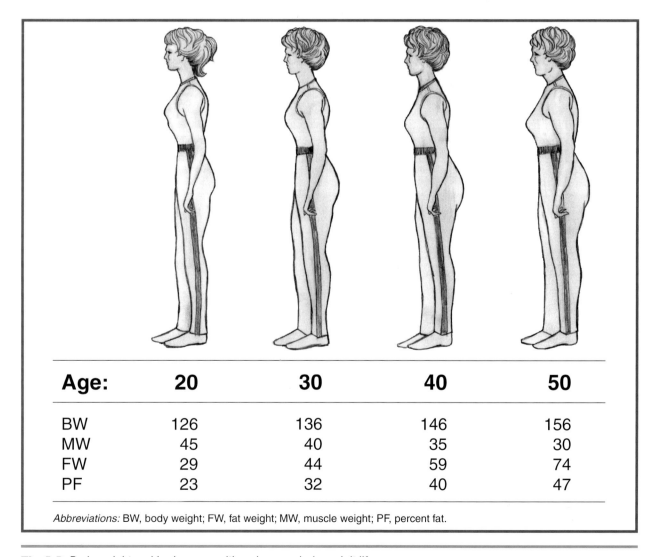

Age:	20	30	40	50
BW	126	136	146	156
MW	45	40	35	30
FW	29	44	59	74
PF	23	32	40	47

Abbreviations: BW, body weight; FW, fat weight; MW, muscle weight; PF, percent fat.

Fig. 2.2 Body weight and body composition changes during adult life.

with either dieting (4-5) or endurance exercise (6) to lose weight more easily. In just eight weeks of Nautilus strength training combined with standard endurance exercise, both younger and senior adults reduced fat weight and increased lean weight, achieving desirable changes in body composition (see table 2.1). These are impressive results for both groups, especially considering that seniors trained only 25 minutes for each type of exercise, two days a week, and younger adults trained the same session duration, just three days a week. And by adding new muscle tissue, strength training increases our energy requirements, or metabolism, at rest—as well as during the exercise session.

Unless you are genetically gifted, strength training is unlikely to produce a Ms. Olympia or Mr. America physique. But regular strength exercise can certainly make the difference between soft, unappealing muscles and firm, attractive muscles. Perhaps the most common comment from new strength training participants is how much better they look as a result of their strength exercise.

Table 2.1
Changes in body composition following eight weeks of strength and endurance exercise (398 subjects).

Training group	Lean weight‡	Fat weight‡	Body composition‡
Younger adults (n=282)	+3.0*	−8.5*	11.5
Seniors (n=116)	+2.5*	−4.0*	6.5

* Significant change (p<0.05)
‡ Change in pounds

Resting Metabolism

Because muscle is very active tissue, our loss of muscle as we age leads to a lower energy requirement and a reduced resting metabolic rate. So without strength exercise, our resting metabolism decreases approximately two to five percent per decade (7, 8). In other words, as we age, we burn fewer calories while resting—unless we exercise.

Both endurance and strength exercise increase our metabolic rate while we are training and for a period of time following the activity session (9). But strength exercise also develops muscle tissue and, therefore, increases our resting metabolism.

In a recent study conducted at Tufts University, senior men and women completed a 12-week program of basic strength exercise (10). The strength training program resulted in three pounds more lean (muscle) weight and four pounds less fat weight. Their resting metabolic rate increased by 7 percent, the equivalent of 108 additional calories per day. This finding indicates that each pound of lean (muscle) weight requires *at least* 35 calories a day at rest for tissue maintenance (as opposed to about two calories a day for each pound of fat).

Table 2.2 shows two women who have the same body weights but different body compositions. The more fit woman has approximately five pounds more muscle tissue and uses about 225 more calories a day at rest.

	Body weight‡	Percent fat	Fat weight‡	Lean weight‡	Estimated muscle weight‡	Resting metabolism+
Table 2.2						
The relationship between muscle and metabolism.						
Tracy:	100	30	30	70	35	850*
Tiffany:	100	20	20	80	40	1075*
Difference:	___	10	10	10	5	225

* Data from BioAnalogics Diagnostic Medical Health Systems, Beaverton, Oregon.
‡ In pounds
+ In calories

Because so many factors affect each individual's resting metabolism, it is not possible to determine a *precise* daily calorie use for each pound of muscle tissue. In spite of that, it is clear that strength training increases muscle mass and that more muscle burns more calories all day long for tissue maintenance. It is certainly safe to say that more muscle helps increase our resting metabolic rate. Imagine burning extra calories even while resting!

Physical Capacity

Everything you do requires a certain percentage of your maximum strength. For example, if your maximum biceps strength is 30 pounds, carrying a 25-pound bag of dog food is a relatively difficult task that quickly becomes an all-out effort. But if you increase your maximum biceps strength to 50 pounds, carrying a 25-pound bag of dog food is a relatively easy task, needing only half of your muscular ability.

Even sitting at a desk demands a degree of muscular effort, particularly in your back and neck muscles. In a study of office workers, the participants' neck strength decreased by 30 percent between 9:00 A.M. and 5:00 P.M., even though all they did was sit at their desks all day (1). They did not realize that their neck muscles were working hard to hold up their 15-pound heads for eight hours. No wonder so many office workers experience neck and back fatigue during the late afternoon hours! Because your muscles are the engines of your body, it is important to maintain a strong muscular system—no matter how you spend the rest of your day. Developing a higher level of muscle strength makes it easier to perform all physical activities.

In simplest terms, power is the product of muscle force and movement speed. For example, to hit a golf ball farther, you could develop more muscle force or you could swing the golf club faster.

Strength training done along with stretching exercise may increase both muscle strength and movement speed. In a study of skilled golfers, eight weeks of strengthening and stretching exercises improved their muscle strength by almost 60 percent and increased their club head speed (golf swing) by over 6 percent. So progressive resistance exercise can enhance athletic power by improving movement speed as well as muscle force.

Health Enhancement

Muscle weakness is related to many degenerative diseases and increased injury potential (7). Recent studies have identified many personal health and physical fitness benefits of regular strength exercise. Our muscular condition impacts many of our body systems and significantly affects our ability to function physically.

• **Injury Prevention.** Weak low back muscles are a major factor in low back pain. Considering that almost 80 percent of Americans suffer from low back problems, this is a significant finding. More importantly, back patients in one study reported significantly less back discomfort after just 12 weeks of specific strength exercise for their low back muscles (11).

Our work with high school athletes has produced similar injury prevention results. We strength trained New England's number one women's cross-country team. They performed a circuit of Nautilus machines, three days a week, during their off-seasons. In contrast to the normally high injury rate for female cross-country runners, the strength trained runners experienced only one injury among the 20 participants in four years.

Properly performed strength exercise makes our muscles better shock absorbers and joint stabilizers. By training all of our major muscle groups, we develop a stronger musculoskeletal system and reduce our risk of muscle imbalance and overuse injuries.

• **Bone Mineral Density.** Progressive resistance exercise places stress on both the muscles and the bones. The muscles respond by increasing their fiber size, while the bones respond by increasing their protein and mineral content. Significant increases in hip bone density can occur after just four months of strength exercise (12).

• **Glucose Metabolism.** Our ability to use glucose efficiently is critically important to our health. In fact, poor glucose metabolism is associated with diabetes. Strength training is an effective means for improving our glucose metabolism, increasing glucose uptake 23 percent after only four months of regular strength exercise (13).

• **Gastrointestinal Transit.** The time necessary to move food matter through our intestines has important health implications. Slow gastrointestinal transit time is related to a higher risk of colon cancer. Gastrointestinal transit can be accelerated by 56 percent after just three months of standard strength exercise (14).

• **Cholesterol (blood lipid) Levels.** Although the effect of strength training on cholesterol levels needs further research, studies have demonstrated improved blood lipid profiles after several weeks of regular strength exercise (15-16). Improvements in cholesterol levels have been similar for both endurance exercise and strength exercise.

• **Arthritic Pain.** Sensible strength training may ease the discomfort of both osteoarthritis and rheumatoid arthritis (17). In addition, strength exercise enables people suffering from arthritis to develop stronger muscles, bones, and connective tissue so they can function better.

• **Resting Blood Pressure.** One of the major fears among younger adults and seniors is that strength training will increase their blood pressure. But properly performed strength exercise is not harmful to blood pressure—even during the exercise set (1) (see table 2.3). Strength training alone can reduce resting blood pressure in mildly hypertensive adults (18). And combining strength and endurance exercise may reduce resting blood pressure even more (19).

In addition to providing important physical benefits, sensible strength exercise itself has an extremely low injury rate. It makes good sense to become a regular participant in a well-designed strength training program.

Table 2.3 Changes in resting blood pressure following eight weeks of strength and endurance exercise (263 subjects).		
Age group	**Systolic blood pressure‡**	**Diastolic blood pressure‡**
Younger adults	–5.0*	–3.0*
Seniors	–7.0*	–4.0*

*Significant change (p<0.05)
‡In mmHg

THE MECHANICS OF MUSCULAR MOVEMENT

A working knowledge of muscle structure and function is essential to best understand and apply the training principles for strength development. That is, in order to most effectively work your muscles, you must know how your muscles work.

The Micromechanics of Movement

Muscle is metabolically active tissue that makes up approximately half of your body weight. Muscle tissue is composed of water (about 80 percent) and protein filaments (about 20 percent). Because of their unique ability to slide together and apart, the interactive protein filaments enable your muscles to contract and relax.

Protein Filaments

A muscle is composed of cylindrical fibers that are responsible for force production (see figure 2.3). Each fiber consists of thick protein filaments called myosin and thin protein filaments called actin. The myosin and actin protein filaments are loosely coupled by means of tiny cross-bridges (see figure 2.4). Although the exact mechanism for muscle enlargement

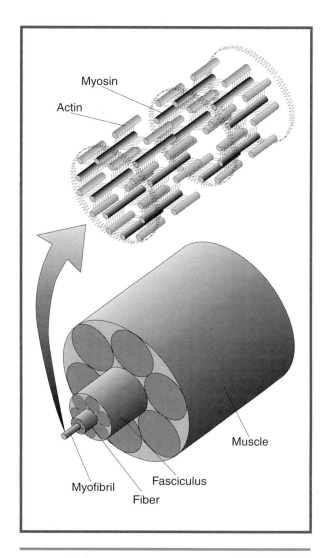

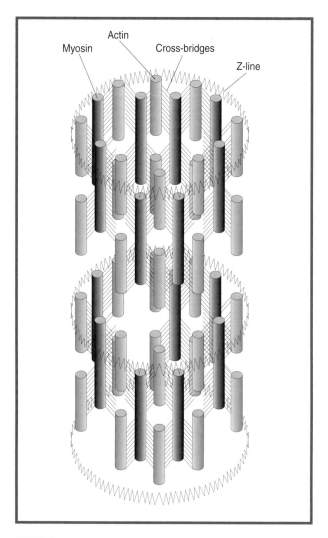

Fig. 2.3 The structural and functional components of skeletal muscle.

Fig. 2.4 Muscle fibers consist of thin actin filaments, thick myosin filaments, and tiny cross-bridges that serve as coupling agents.

is not fully understood, it is believed that progressive strength exercise increases the number or size of the protein filaments, increasing the size of each muscle fiber (see figure 2.5). Strength training leads to larger muscle fibers (hypertrophy), and lack of strength training leads to smaller muscle fibers (atrophy).

Muscle Activation

The sliding action of the actin and myosin protein filaments is caused by electrical, chemical, and mechanical interactions. The electrical stimulus for muscle contraction comes from a motor nerve located in the central nervous system. The motor nerve branches into many nerve endings, each of which attaches to a different muscle fiber. The motor nerve and all of the muscle fibers it serves form a system known as the motor unit (see figure 2.6). The electrical stimulus from the central nervous system reaches all of the attached muscle fibers at the same instant,

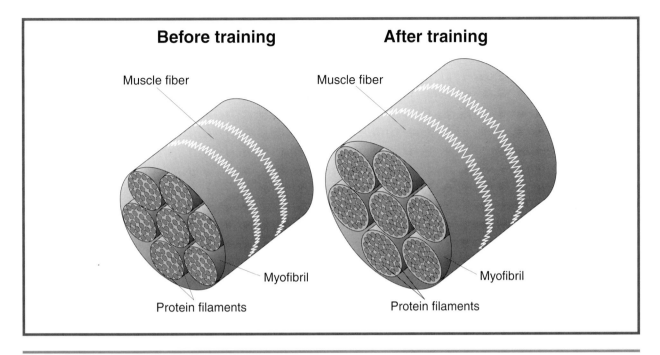

Fig. 2.5 Possible mechanism for enlarging muscle fiber size.

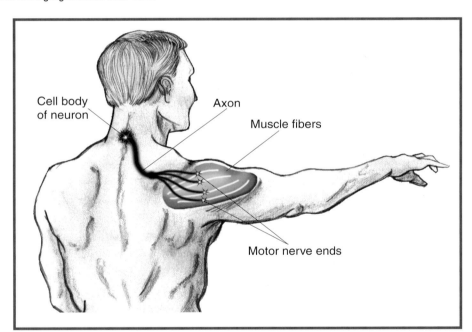

Fig. 2.6 The motor unit consists of a single motor nerve and all of the muscle fibers that it innervates.

causing them to contract with maximum force. Because the muscle fibers in a given motor unit are evenly distributed throughout the muscle, their simultaneous activation produces a smooth muscle contraction.

The chemical stimulus for muscle contraction is the splitting of a compound substance called ATP into its component parts. This chemical change releases energy that enables the actin and myosin protein filaments to slide together and produce movement.

The mechanical interactions responsible for muscle contraction occur when the thin actin protein filaments slide between the thick myosin protein filaments. Just like interlocking your finger tips and sliding your hands together, the interactions between the actin and myosin protein filaments produce friction that affects your muscle force output.

Muscle Relaxation

Muscle relaxation is a passive process. When the electrical stimulus from the central nervous system stops, the sliding interactions between the actin and myosin protein filaments also stop and the muscle relaxes. When the muscle on one side of a joint contracts, the muscle on the other side of the joint must relax. For example, when your biceps contracts and shortens, your triceps relaxes and lengthens. The simultaneous contraction and relaxation of opposite muscles permits smooth and productive movement.

The Mechanics of Movement and Resistance Exercise

Muscle action initiates every movement we make. The more resistance we have to move, the more muscle force we need to use.

Muscle Contraction

An activated muscle produces force that lifts, lowers, or holds resistance. During a positive (concentric) contraction, the muscle exerts force, shortens, and overcomes the resistance. For example, your biceps perform a positive contraction when lifting a barbell from your hips to your shoulders.

During a negative (eccentric) contraction, the muscle exerts force, lengthens, and is overcome by the resistance. For example, your biceps perform a negative contraction when lowering a barbell from your shoulders to your hips.

During a static (isometric) contraction, the muscle exerts force but does not change length. It neither overcomes nor is overcome by the resistance, but simply maintains a specific position. For example, your biceps perform a static contraction when holding a barbell at a right angle. Keep in mind that all three muscle contractions (positive, negative, and static) require energy and produce force.

Muscle Force Output

Your muscle force output is affected by friction between the actin and myosin protein filaments as they slide together and apart. Friction always opposes the direction of movement. During a positive contraction, friction opposes muscle shortening, which decreases your muscle force output by about 20 percent. During a negative contraction friction opposes muscle lengthening, which increases your muscle force output by about 20 percent.

Let's assume that your biceps can produce 100 pounds of force and that you can briefly hold (static contraction) a 100-pound barbell at a right angle (see figure 2.7c). Because static contractions do not involve

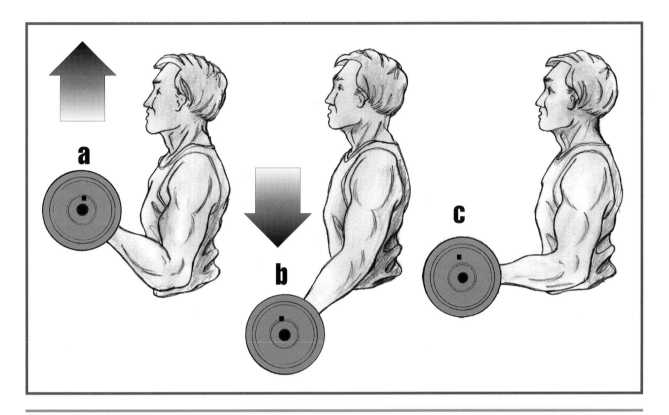

Fig. 2.7 (a) Positive contraction of the biceps lifting an 80-pound barbell; (b) negative contraction of the biceps lowering a 120-pound barbell; and (c) static contraction of the biceps holding a 100-pound barbell.

friction, your muscle force output (100 pounds) is essentially the same as your muscle force input (100 pounds).

You discover, however, that you can slowly lift (positive contraction) only an 80-pound barbell from your hips to your shoulders (see figure 2.7a). Although your muscle force input is still 100 pounds, friction subtracts 20 pounds, or 20 percent, for a positive muscle force output of only 80 pounds.

Next, you discover that you can slowly lower (negative contraction) a 120-pound barbell from your shoulders to your hips (see figure 2.7b). Although your muscle force input is still 100 pounds, friction adds 20 pounds, or 20 percent, for a negative muscle force output of 120 pounds. Try this yourself, and you will discover that you can lower much more weight than you can lift. So you should perform your lowering movements more slowly than your lifting movements to make the negative muscle contractions more challenging and productive.

Prime Mover, Antagonistic, and Stabilizer Muscles

The muscles primarily responsible for a given joint movement are called the prime mover muscles. The prime mover muscles contract positively during lifting movements and contract negatively during lowering movements. For example, your biceps are the prime mover muscles for both the lifting phase and the lowering phase of barbell curls.

The muscles primarily responsible for the opposing joint movement are known as antagonist muscles. Your triceps are the antagonists of your biceps for both the lifting phase and the lowering phase of barbell curls.

Muscles that maintain desired body positions are referred to as stabilizer muscles. In order for your biceps to perform a barbell curl, several other muscle groups must contract in a static position to stabilize your torso and upper arms. For example, your low back muscles must contract in a static position to keep your torso erect, and your pectoralis major and latissimus dorsi must contract in a static position to secure your upper arms against your sides. These muscle groups function, therefore, as stabilizers while you perform barbell curls.

Fiber Types

As discussed in chapter 1, our muscles are composed of two basic fiber types, known as slow-twitch (type I) and fast-twitch (type II). During strength exercise, the smaller slow-twitch muscle fibers are activated before the larger fast-twitch muscle fibers. However, the less-enduring fast-twitch fibers fatigue sooner than the more-enduring slow-twitch fibers.

As a hypothetical example of muscle fiber involvement, consider figure 2.8. Assume that you have 10 biceps fibers, 5 of which are slow-twitch and 5 of which are fast-twitch. Assume that each slow-twitch fiber can produce four pounds of force and that each fast-twitch fiber can produce five pounds of force. Assume that each slow-twitch fiber can endure 12 repetitions and that each fast-twitch fiber can endure 2 repetitions.

Now begin a set of 25-pound dumbbell curls. To produce 25 pounds of muscle force, you activate all 5 slow-twitch fibers (20 pounds of force) first, followed by 1 fast-twitch fiber (5 pounds of force). After two repetitions, the first fast-twitch fiber fatigues and a fresh fast-twitch fiber re-

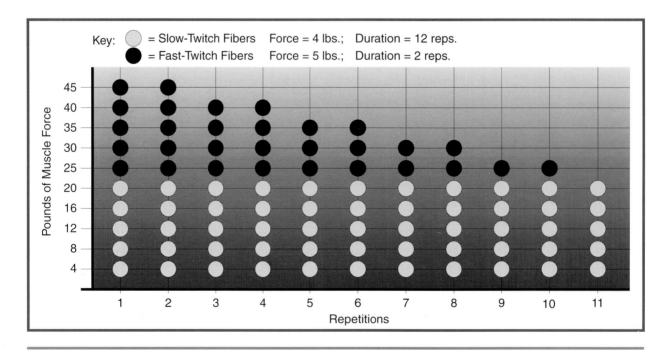

Fig. 2.8 Hypothetical example of muscle fiber involvement during a 10-repetition set of 25-pound dumbbell curls.

places it. After two more repetitions, the second fast-twitch fiber fatigues and a fresh fast-twitch fiber replaces it. After two more repetitions, the third fast-twitch fiber fatigues and a fresh fast-twitch fiber replaces it. After two more repetitions the fourth fast-twitch fiber fatigues and a fresh fast-twitch fiber replaces it. After two more repetitions, the last fast-twitch fiber fatigues, leaving only 20 pounds of force from the more-enduring slow-twitch fibers. Of course, this is not sufficient force to lift 25 pounds of resistance, so you must end the exercise set after 10 repetitions. If, after resting, you perform a second set of dumbbell curls, you will activate the same muscle fibers in the same order as the first set.

Motor Unit

A motor unit consists of a single motor nerve and all of the muscle fibers that it activates. When the motor unit is activated, all of the muscle fibers contract at the same instant with maximum force. Slow-twitch motor units are smaller and include an average of 100 slow-twitch muscle fibers. Fast-twitch motor units are larger and include an average of 500 fast-twitch muscle fibers. Lifting a light (10-pound) dumbbell requires only a few motor units (slow-twitch) and many repetitions are possible. Lifting a heavy (50-pound) dumbbell requires many motor units (slow-twitch and fast-twitch) and few repetitions are possible (see figure 2.9).

During the early stages of strength training, much of the performance improvement is due to better motor unit selection. This process, known as "motor learning," identifies and preferentially activates the most effective motor units for a given exercise.

Muscle Fatigue

Many physiological factors may contribute to momentary muscle fatigue. One possible cause is interference with electrical impulses, particularly where the nerve endings and muscle fibers meet. Another source of muscle

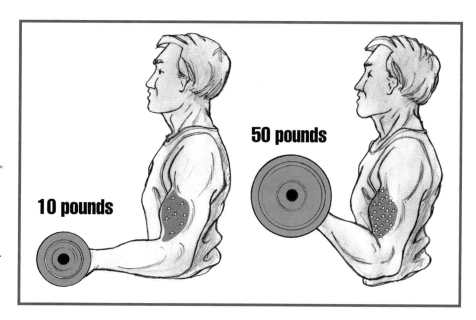

Fig. 2.9 Few motor units (slow-twitch) are activated to lift a 10-pound dumbbell, and many motor units (slow-twitch and fast-twitch) are activated to lift a 50-pound dumbbell.

fatigue may be the temporary depletion of chemical energy sources (ATP). But the most likely fatigue factor is the accumulation of lactic acid within the muscle. Excess lactic acid increases tissue acidity, which probably activates pain sensors. Whatever the underlying causes may be, the discomfort is temporary and passes quickly after the exercise set. Momentary muscle fatigue should not deter you from a well-designed strength training program.

Muscle Soreness

Muscle discomfort that occurs a day or two after your workout is referred to as delayed onset muscle soreness (DOMS). It is typically associated with new movement patterns and negative muscle contractions. DOMS most likely results from microscopic tears within the muscle fibers. Light tissue microtrauma usually requires two or three recovery days for building processes that lead to larger and stronger muscles. Heavy tissue microtrauma, however, may require several recovery days for repair processes that do not necessarily result in larger and stronger muscles. So you should train in a sensible and systematic manner, avoiding excessively hard exercise sessions.

TYPES OF EXERCISE

You may exercise your muscles differently, depending on the type of resistance you use in your training program. Safety and effectiveness should be the key factors in selecting your exercise mode.

Isometric Exercise

Isometric exercise involves static muscle contractions done against a stationary resistance. Isometric exercise effectively builds muscle strength, but its lack of movement is associated with certain training problems. First, isometric exercise increases muscle strength only in the joint positions used. To develop full-range muscle strength with isometrics, it is necessary to train at several positions throughout the movement range.

Second, static muscle contractions tend to block blood flow, which may produce unsafe blood pressure responses. For this reason, older individuals and persons with cardiovascular problems should avoid isometric forms of exercise.

Third, most people have difficulty assessing their exercise effort and training progress with isometric strengthening programs. The lack of movement makes monotony and motivation serious obstacles to regular isometric training.

Isokinetic Exercise

Although there are a few exceptions, isokinetic exercise generally involves only positive muscle contractions against an accommodating hydraulic or electronic resistance. The training device maintains a constant movement speed, and the muscle force you give determines the resistance force you receive. That is, if you give low muscle force, you receive low resistance force, and if you give high muscle force, you receive high resistance force. For example, when swimming, if you give a low-effort arm stroke, you encounter low resistance from the water, but if you give a high-effort arm stroke, you encounter high resistance from the water. Therefore, isokinetic resistance is somewhat "soft." If you inadvertently give less muscle effort, you automatically encounter less resistance, and so gain fewer benefits.

Isotonic Exercise

Isotonic exercise has several differences in comparison with isokinetic exercise. First, isotonic exercise includes both positive and negative muscle contractions. Second, isotonic exercise does not require a constant movement speed. For example, you may lift the barbell in two seconds and lower the barbell in four seconds. Third, you control your effort level by selecting a certain resistance force and your muscles must respond accordingly. In other words, the more resistance you select the more muscle force you need to perform each repetition.

Isotonic exercise may be performed with a constant resistance or with a variable resistance. Although the same principles apply, each type of resistance has a different pattern of muscle force production.

Dynamic Constant Resistance Exercise

This form of isotonic exercise uses a fixed resistance, such as a barbell. Although the resistance does not change, your muscle force is lower in some positions and higher in other positions due to leverage factors. As shown in figure 2.10, the barbell provides 100 pounds of resistance force throughout the pressing movement, even though the muscle force increases from 100 pounds in the bottom position to 140 pounds in the top position because of movement mechanics. Consequently, dynamic constant resistance exercise may provide a poor matching of muscle force and resistance force throughout the movement range.

Dynamic Variable Resistance Exercise

As the name implies, this form of isotonic exercise uses a resistance that automatically changes throughout the movement range. For example, Nautilus machines incorporate a cam to automatically vary the resistance, matching your muscle force pattern. That is, you encounter proportionately less resistance in positions of lower muscle force and proportionately more resistance in positions of higher muscle force. The Nautilus machine smoothly increases the resistance from 100 pounds in the bottom position to 140 pounds in the top position (see figure 2.11). This results in a better matching of muscle force and resistance force throughout the movement range, which makes dynamic variable resistance exercise a more productive means of strength training.

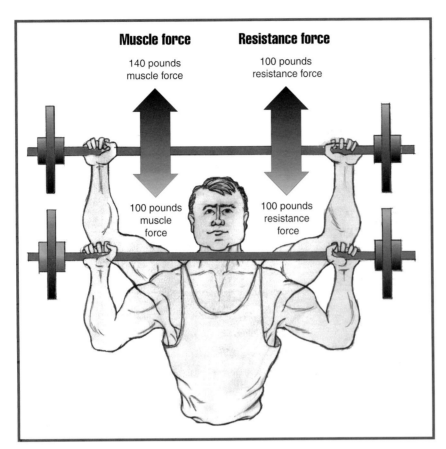

Fig. 2.10 Dynamic constant resistance exercise may provide a poor matching of muscle force and resistance force.

SUMMARY

Sensible strength training provides many health and fitness benefits related to muscle development. Fitness benefits include improved muscle strength, muscle endurance, cardiovascular endurance, joint flexibility, body composition, resting metabolism, and physical capacity. Health factors benefiting from strength training include improved bone mineral density, glucose metabolism, gastrointestinal transit, cholesterol levels, resting blood pressure, and reduced arthritic pain.

Your muscles consist of water and protein filaments which adapt well to progressive resistance exercise. When stimulated by a nerve impulse, the protein filaments slide together to produce a muscle contraction. The muscle contracts positively to perform lifting movements and negatively to perform lowering movements. Your muscles consist of two types of fibers, known as slow-twitch and fast-twitch. Slow-twitch muscle fibers produce lower force levels for longer periods, while fast-twitch muscle fibers produce higher force levels for shorter periods.

Because of leverage factors, your muscle force is higher in some positions and lower in other positions. Dynamic variable resistance exercise automatically changes the resistance force to match your muscle force throughout the movement range. When training with proper exercise technique and intensity, this is the most effective way to maximize your strength development.

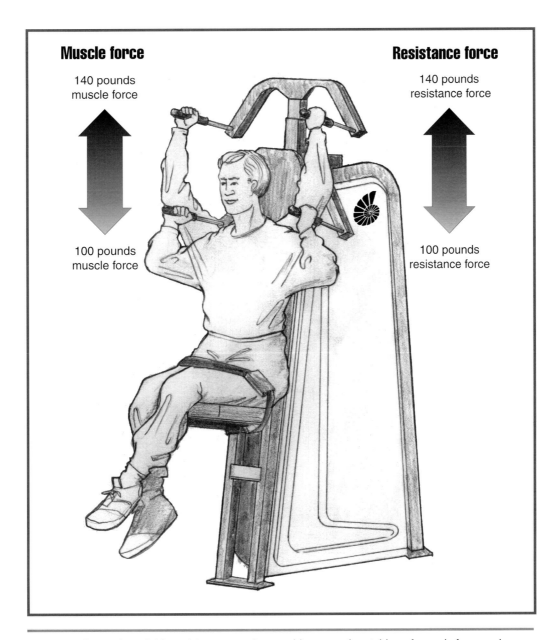

Muscle force

140 pounds
muscle force

100 pounds
muscle force

Resistance force

140 pounds
resistance force

100 pounds
resistance force

Fig. 2.11 Dynamic variable resistance exercise provides a good matching of muscle force and resistance force due to the cam, which automatically changes resistance force.

CHAPTER 3

Training Your Muscles

Now that you know how your muscles work, you'll want to know how to work your muscles safely. Although there are many different training programs for increasing muscle strength, some pose a high risk of injury, while others require a major time commitment. What you need is a program that has been thoroughly tested for safe, effective, and efficient strength development.

BASIC STRENGTH TRAINING GUIDELINES

Although relatively simple in concept, the following procedures are so productive that many professional football teams follow them.

Exercise Selection and Order

A sound strength training program should include exercises for all of your major muscle groups. If you select your exercises carefully, your muscles will develop in balance with each other and you'll have a firm foundation for further improvement. For example, you should not emphasize some muscle groups over others because this can result in muscle imbalance injuries. When I was a university track coach, I had my sprinters perform strengthening exercises for their quadriceps and stretching exercises for their hamstrings. This procedure produced relatively strong quadriceps and relatively weak hamstrings, which set the stage for hamstring injuries. I soon learned the importance of a comprehensive training program to develop overall muscle strength and to reduce the risk of injury.

Do your best to exercise your larger muscle groups first, followed by your medium and smaller muscle groups. For example, you may begin with your legs, then work on your torso, arms, midsection, and neck. You should also try to pair your exercises, working opposing muscle groups in succession.

Table 3.1 shows the Nautilus machines that best address the major and minor muscles in general order of larger to smaller groups, with opposing muscle groups paired.

Frequency

Properly performed strength exercise progressively stresses your muscles and produces some degree of tissue microtrauma. Following your training session, the stressed tissue undergoes repair and building processes

Table 3.1
Muscles and exercises in general order from larger to smaller muscle groups.

Major muscle groups	Appropriate Nautilus machines
Quadriceps	Leg extension, leg press
Hamstrings	Seated leg curl, prone leg curl, leg press
Hip adductors	Hip adductor
Hip abductors	Hip abductor
Pectoralis major	10° chest, 50° chest, chest cross, decline press, incline press, bench press, chin-dip
Latissimus dorsi	Super pullover, behind-the-neck, torso arm, compound row, chin-dip
Deltoids	Lateral raise, rowing back, rotary shoulder, overhead press
Biceps	Preacher curl, chin-dip
Triceps	Triceps extension, chin-dip, seated dip
Low back	Low back
Abdominals	Abdominal
Neck	4-way neck

Minor muscle groups	
Obliques	Rotary torso
Upper trapezius	Neck and shoulder
Hip flexors	Lower abdominal
Calves	Seated calf
Forearms	Super-forearm

that lead to larger and stronger muscles. Your muscles usually need between 48 and 72 hours to complete these physiological changes, and each new workout should take place at the peak of this muscle-building process. Unfortunately, the only way to determine your most productive recovery and building period is through trial and error. That's why it's so important to maintain a detailed record of each training session. If your exercise frequency is appropriate, you should notice some strength improvements every workout.

Generally speaking, two or three strength training sessions a week produce excellent results for most people (1). Two strength workouts a week are 75 percent as productive as three strength workouts a week (1-3). Table 3.2 summarizes research on two versus three days a week of strength training. It shows that two-days-a-week participants gained about 75 percent as much muscle strength and lean weight as three-days-a-week participants.

Based on this research, you should aim for three strength training sessions a week.

Table 3.2 Comparison of two and three training sessions per week on muscle strength and mass (81 subjects).		
8 weeks of training	**2 days/week**	**3 days/week**
Muscle strength (percent) (33 subjects)	+17.0	+24.0
Muscle mass (pounds) (48 subjects)	+3.0	+3.9

But if that's just too much for your schedule, remember that in two days, you can still get 75 percent as much benefit as in three days. Two days are great compared to none, so don't let a lack of time prevent you from training.

Perhaps as important as your exercise frequency is your training consistency. Try to stay on your training schedule and avoid back-to-back strength workouts. For example, it's not a good idea to train only one day a week, and it is usually counterproductive to work the same muscles two days in a row.

Sets

In 1990, the American College of Sports Medicine recommended one or more sets per workout of resistance exercise for strength development (4). While it is obvious that you must perform at least one set of strength work, most people are unaware that additional sets may have little extra value. Similar strength benefits can come from single-set and multiple-set strength training. For example, researchers examined strength gains in 77 subjects who did one, two, or three sets of upper body exercise over a 10-week training period (5). All three exercise groups made similar improvements in upper body muscle strength (see figure 3.1).

Other researchers compared strength gains in 38 subjects who performed one or three sets of lower body exercise over a 14-week training period (6). Both exercise groups experienced similar improvements in

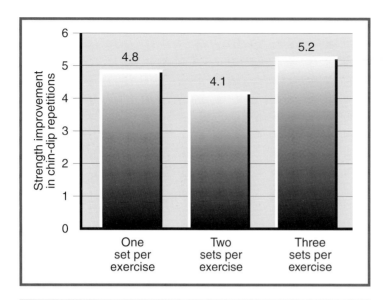

Fig. 3.1 Comparison of one-, two-, and three-set strength training (77 subjects).

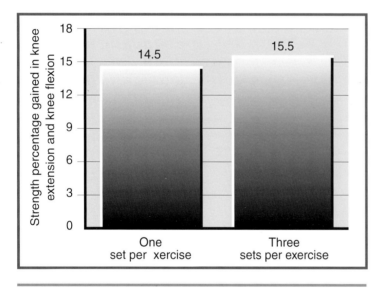

Fig. 3.2 Comparison of one- and three-set strength training (38 subjects).

lower body muscle strength (see figure 3.2), increasing their knee extension and knee flexion strength by about 15 percent.

You can see that one properly performed exercise set is as effective for increasing muscle strength as two or three exercise sets. Because single-set training is more time-efficient than multiple-set training, and because many people live on tight schedules, you should perform one good set of each exercise. Single-set training is a safe, effective, and efficient means for developing muscle strength.

Exercise Resistance

For decades, the overload principle has been the key concept in strength training. "Overloading" means using progressively heavier resistance to work the muscles harder, encouraging further strength development. For example, if you can curl 100 pounds one time, then one repetition with 105 pounds will overload your biceps. Or if you can curl 50 pounds your biceps. Or if you can curl 50 pounds 20 times, then 20 repetitions with 55 pounds would also overload your biceps.

Using a relatively high resistance increases your chances for injury, while doing a relatively high number of repetitions decreases your strength benefits. So what are the best guidelines for applying the overload principle?

Muscle strength may be best developed by working the target muscle to fatigue within the anaerobic energy system. This is the system that supplies energy for high-effort exercise lasting less than 90 seconds. For most practical purposes, about 50 to 70 seconds of continuous resistance exercise to the point of muscle fatigue is preferred. Most people can perform about 50 to 70 seconds of strength work with 75 percent of their maximum resistance. At a moderate speed (six seconds a repetition) this corresponds to 8 to 12 controlled repetitions.

Fortunately, you can estimate 75 percent of your maximum resistance without doing an all-out lift. Simply find the weight that you can do 10 times to fatigue and this should be about 75 percent of your maximum. Training with three-fourths of maximum resistance creates a high strength stimulus and poses a low risk of injury. While 75 percent of maximum resistance is standard strength training procedure, periodically training with lower and higher percentages of your maximum resistance offers you a welcome change of pace, giving you both physiological and psychological benefits.

Repetitions

An inverse relationship exists between the amount of resistance we use and the number of repetitions we can perform. That is, you can perform fewer repetitions with a relatively heavy resistance and more repetitions with a relatively light resistance.

Another less obvious factor influences the number of repetitions you can complete with a given resistance. If you have inherited predominantly fast-twitch muscle fibers, you will have lower muscle endurance and perform fewer repetitions than average with a specific resistance. If you have inherited predominantly slow-twitch muscle fibers, you will have higher muscle endurance and perform more repetitions than average with a specific resistance.

To learn more about repetitions, a study was conducted of 141 subjects who had been using the same training procedures (7). The first step was to determine the maximum resistance that each participant could perform for one repetition. The second step was to discover how many repetitions each participant could complete with 75 percent of his or her maximum resistance.

Most of the subjects completed between 8 and 12 repetitions with 75 percent of their maximum resistance (see figure 3.3). At six seconds a repetition, these subjects experienced muscle fatigue in 50 to 70 seconds of continuous muscle effort. They were average individuals who had moderate muscle endurance, most likely due to an even mix of fast-twitch and slow-twitch muscle fibers.

Notice that some of the participants performed fewer than eight repetitions with 75 percent of their maximum resistance. These individuals were power athletes (sprinters) who had low muscle endurance, probably because of a greater percentage of fast-twitch muscle fibers. At six seconds a repetition, these subjects experienced muscle fatigue within approximately 30 to 50 seconds of continuous exercise.

At the other extreme, a few of the participants performed more than 12 repetitions with 75 percent of their maximum resistance. They were endurance athletes (e.g., distance runners) who had high muscle endurance, probably because of a greater percentage of slow-twitch muscle fibers. At six seconds a repetition, these subjects experienced muscle fatigue within approximately 70 to 90 seconds of continuous exercise, still within the anaerobic energy system.

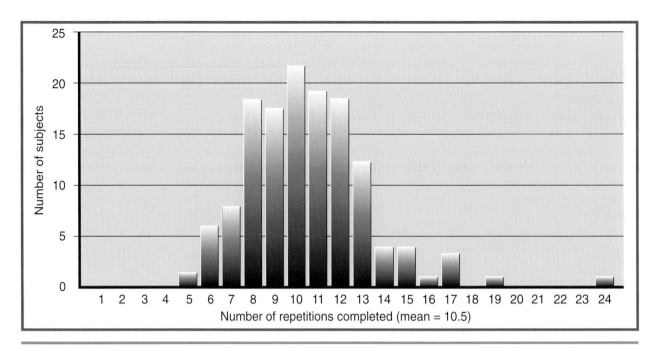

Fig. 3.3 Distribution of repetitions completed with 75 percent of maximum weight load (141 subjects).

Based on these findings and follow-up research that matched the exercise duration to each individual's muscle endurance, the following repetition guidelines are recommended. People with low-endurance muscles generally gain better results by training with about five to eight repetitions (30 to 50 seconds) a set. People with moderate-endurance muscles generally gain better results by training with about 8 to 12 repetitions (50 to 70 seconds) a set. People with high-endurance muscles generally gain better results by training with about 12 to 15 repetitions (70 to 90 seconds) a set.

Because most people have moderate-endurance muscles, 8 to 12 repetitions a set are suggested as standard training procedure. Still, you may periodically perform greater or fewer repetitions a set for a change of pace.

Progression

Continued strength development depends on progressive resistance exercise that gradually places more stress on the target muscles. A double-progressive training system, in which you alternately add repetitions and resistance, is preferred. For example, maybe you can do eight lateral raises with 50 pounds. Continue training with 50 pounds until you can do 12 repetitions. Then increase the resistance by about 5 percent. That is, add two and one-half pounds to the weight stack and train with 52.5 pounds until you can again do 12 repetitions.

By systematically increasing the exercise repetitions up to twelve, then increasing the exercise resistance by 5 percent, you ensure gradual strength gains with the lowest risk of injury. Although there are other workout programs, this system fatigues the target muscles within 50 to 70 seconds of continuous exercise, which is the best anaerobic training range for most people.

Speed

Exercise speed may be divided into three categories: fast, moderate, and slow. A fast exercise speed is one that you cannot stop. Fast exercise speed emphasizes momentum, which reduces muscle effort and increases the risk of injury. Lifting movements under two seconds qualify as fast.

A moderate exercise speed is one that you can stop. Moderate exercise speed de-emphasizes momentum, increasing muscle effort and reducing the risk of injury. Lifting movements between two and four seconds are of moderate speed.

A slow exercise speed is one that you completely control. Slow exercise speed minimizes momentum and maximizes muscle tension. Lifting movements over four seconds are slow.

Let's look at a study that examined different exercise speeds (8). The 198 subjects were divided into four training groups (see table 3.3). Group A did 4-second repetitions (2 seconds lifting and 2 seconds lowering). Group B did 6-second repetitions (2 seconds lifting and 4 seconds lowering). Group C did 8-second repetitions (4 seconds lifting and 4 seconds lowering). Group D did 14-second repetitions (10 seconds lifting and 4 seconds lowering). All of the training groups completed their exercise sets within the anaerobic energy system (less than 90 seconds).

Table 3.3			
Eight-week improvements in muscle strength using different movement speeds (198 subjects).			
8-week program (seconds per rep)	Reps per set	Time per set (seconds)	Mean weight increase 13 Nautilus machines (pounds)
A. 4	10	40	22
B. 6	10	60	22
C. 8	10	80	23
D. 14	5	70	27

Although the slower exercise speeds produced slightly better results, all of the moderate to slow exercise speeds were effective for increasing muscle strength during the eight-week training period.

Moderate to slow exercise speeds have the following training advantages over fast exercise speeds:

1. A longer period of muscle tension
2. A higher level of muscle force
3. A lower level of momentum
4. A lower risk of tissue injury

Six-second repetitions, with two seconds for the lifting movements and four seconds for the lowering movements, are preferred. The longer lowering phase causes a more productive negative muscle contraction. While six-second repetitions are considered standard training procedure, using other moderate-to-slow movement speeds is acceptable.

Range

You should perform full-range exercise movements to develop full-range muscle strength. This is because muscle strength is somewhat specific to the movement range that is trained. For example, back extensions performed in one-half of the movement range have their greatest strengthening effect in that area (9).

Full-range muscle strength is especially important for low back patients. People who have little strength in the position of full-trunk extension are more likely to experience low back pain. Fortunately, strength training the low back muscles through their full movement range can significantly reduce pain (10).

Because full-range muscle strength enhances physical performance and reduces the risk of injury, you should perform full-range resistance exercise whenever possible. Although the range of joint movement varies among individuals, you should train from the position of full muscle stretch to the position of full muscle contraction. Keep in mind that when the target muscle (e.g., biceps) is fully contracted, the opposing muscle (e.g., triceps) is fully stretched. For this reason, full-range resistance training may enhance joint flexibility as well as increase muscle strength (3).

Activity Order

You should do strength exercise to improve your muscular fitness and endurance exercise to improve your cardiovascular fitness. You may begin your workout, though, with either exercise because you can achieve similar strength gains regardless of the activity order (11).

For example, 43 participants did 20 minutes of strength exercise and 20 minutes of endurance exercise, three days a week for eight weeks (2). They used 10 different Nautilus machines for strength training and did cycling, walking, and stepping for endurance training. Half of the subjects always did their strength exercise first, and half always did their endurance exercise first. Both training groups experienced virtually equal strength gains after eight weeks of exercise (see table 3.4).

Do the activity that is most important to you first. For example, if your primary goal is muscular fitness, you should do the strength exercise first. If your main objective is cardiovascular fitness, you should do the endurance exercise first.

Table 3.4
Changes in muscle strength for subjects who did strength training first and subjects who did endurance training first (43 subjects).

8-week training program	Mean weight increase, 11 Nautilus machines (pounds)
Strength exercise first	22
Endurance exercise first	23

Whichever type of activity order you prefer to start with, begin each training session with a few minutes of warm-up exercise and end with a few minutes of cool-down exercise. These transition phases between rest and vigorous physical activity may provide important physiological and psychological benefits. Easy walking and cycling are appropriate activities for warming up and cooling down.

Breathing

Breathe continuously while performing strength exercise. Regardless of the exercise effort, you should never hold your breath. The internal pressure caused by holding your breath coupled with the external pressure of forceful muscle contractions may limit blood flow to your brain and heart. To avoid light-headedness and high blood pressure, breathe continuously throughout every exercise set.

Exhale during lifting movements and inhale during lowering movements. This decreases the internal air pressure as the external muscular pressure increases and vice versa.

Intensity

High-intensity exercise enhances strength development (4). Your exercise effort should be hard enough to fatigue the target muscles within the anaerobic energy system (about 50 to 70 seconds). This typically requires 8 to 12 repetitions with 75 percent of your maximum resistance. For best results, use moderate to slow exercise speed, full-range movement, and correct performance technique.

HIGH-INTENSITY TRAINING

One way to make your workout more demanding is to perform more sets and more exercises. Bodybuilders have traditionally taken this approach, training two to four hours a day, six days a week. But recently, because of time limitations and overtraining injuries, many strength enthusiasts have taken a different approach to advanced training. Called high-intensity strength training, it has produced excellent results for champion bodybuilders and professional football teams.

The basic premise of high-intensity strength training is to put more effort into each exercise set rather than to perform more sets. This type of training emphasizes the exercise intensity instead of the exercise duration. Because the motor unit activation pattern is the same for a given exercise, multiple-set training fatigues the same muscle fibers again and again.

For example, if you perform 10 leg extensions to temporary muscle failure with 75 percent of your maximum resistance, you fatigue 25 percent of your quadriceps fibers. If you rest two minutes and repeat this procedure, you again fatigue 25 percent of your quadriceps fibers. You have just stimulated the same 25 percent of your quadriceps fibers once again.

In contrast, let's say you perform 10 leg extensions to temporary muscle failure with 75 percent of your maximum resistance, which fatigues 25

Summary of Strength Training Principles

For a safe, sensible, and successful strength training experience, use these basic principles of muscle conditioning.

Exercise Selection and Order

Perform strength training exercises for all of your major muscle groups, beginning with the larger muscles of your legs and progressing to the smaller muscles of your torso, arms, mid-section, and neck.

Exercise Frequency

Follow a training frequency of three days a week, with 48 to 72 hours rest between exercise sessions for the muscle rebuilding processes to take place. Two strength workouts a week provide almost as much muscle-building benefit as three strength workouts a week and is an effective training alternative.

Sets

Similar strength gains come from one, two, and three sets of resistance exercise. Because single-set training is more efficient than multiple-set training, do one good set of each exercise.

Resistance

Develop muscle strength by working the target muscle to fatigue within the anaerobic energy system (50 to 70 seconds), usually training with about 75 percent of your maximum resistance.

Repetitions

Most people can complete about 8 to 12 repetitions with 75 percent of their maximum resistance. At six seconds a repetition, this requires about 50 to 70 seconds of continuous muscle effort and is highly productive.

Progression

Increase the training resistance by about 5 percent whenever you can complete 12 repetitions. This gradual training approach makes sure that the exercise resistance will fatigue the target muscles within the anaerobic energy system.

Speed

Moderate to slow exercise speeds are safe and effective for strength development. Because it has a long history of success, do six seconds a repetition, with two seconds for each lifting movement and four seconds for each lowering movement.

Range

Whenever possible, perform strength exercise through a full range of joint movement. Full-range resistance exercise does a better job of strengthening the target muscles and of stretching the opposing muscles.

Order

Whether you perform strength or endurance exercise first is a matter of personal preference. Whichever activity order you choose, begin each training session with a warm-up and end with a cool-down.

Breathing

Be sure to breathe continuously while performing strength exercise. Exhale during the lifting movements and inhale during the lowering movements.

Intensity

Perhaps the most important component of successful strength training is the exercise intensity. High-intensity exercise requires you to fatigue the target muscles within the anaerobic energy system (50 to 70 seconds). For best results, couple high training effort with correct performance technique.

percent of your quadriceps fibers. Instead of stopping, you quickly reduce the resistance and perform a few additional repetitions. By immediately completing a few post-failure repetitions with a lighter resistance, you fatigue more muscle fibers. That is, you experience two levels of muscle failure within the same extended exercise set, providing a greater stimulus for strength development.

Breakdown Training

You now know that one means for fatiguing more muscle fibers is to perform a few additional repetitions with slightly less resistance as soon as you reach temporary muscle failure. This high-intensity technique is called breakdown training, because you break down the resistance to accommodate your momentarily reduced muscle strength.

As a general rule, go to temporary muscle failure with your standard resistance, then quickly reduce the resistance about 10 to 20 percent. This should permit you to complete two to four additional repetitions, reaching a second level of muscle failure within the anaerobic energy system (under 90 seconds).

Researchers recently examined the effects of breakdown training on strength development (12). All 45 adult subjects performed standard training (one set of 8 to 12 repetitions) on 11 Nautilus machines for the

General Guidelines for High-Intensity Training

High-intensity strength training is an effective and efficient means for overcoming strength plateaus, stimulating further muscle development. Instead of increasing the exercise duration by doing more sets, this approach increases the exercise intensity by performing harder sets.

Because you cannot train very hard for very long, keep high-intensity strength sessions relatively brief. I recommend no more than 20 minutes of high-intensity training, including no more than 10 different exercises.

Because high-intensity workouts require more recovery time for tissue building, you should perform them only once or twice a week. If you prefer to do more frequent high-intensity training, consider emphasizing different body parts on different days. For example, during one workout you might perform standard training for the legs and high-intensity training for the upper body. During the next workout you might perform standard training for the upper body and high-intensity training for the legs.

For better results combine your high-intensity training with plenty of rest and proper nutrition. It is especially important to stay well-hydrated, so drink several glasses of water or juice every day.

first four weeks of the study. During the second four weeks, half of the subjects continued their standard training, while the other half performed breakdown training on two of the machines (seated leg curl and abdominal). The participants who performed breakdown training experienced over 30 percent more strength development during the eight-week exercise period (see table 3.5). The standard training produced an 18-pound improvement in the two exercises, while the breakdown training produced a 25-pound improvement. Breakdown training is clearly an effective and efficient means for increasing muscle strength. And because it always reduces the starting resistance, breakdown training is also a safe exercise technique.

Table 3.5
Comparison of standard and breakdown training (45 subjects).

8-week training program	Mean weight increase, 2 Nautilus machines (pounds)
Standard training	18
Breakdown training	25

Assisted Training

Another high-intensity training procedure for fatiguing more muscle fibers is known as assisted training. Like breakdown training, assisted training allows you to complete a few additional repetitions with reduced resistance when you reach temporary muscle failure. In assisted training, however, the weight on the machine remains the same. When you cannot do another repetition, your training partner gives you just enough assistance to lift the resistance (see figure 3.4). Because your muscles are stronger in negative contractions, your training partner does not assist you during the lowering movements.

But as you further fatigue your target muscles, the negative contractions become increasingly more difficult. At the point where you can no longer control the lowering movement, end the extended exercise set. Generally speaking, this will occur within two to four assisted repetitions. With assisted training, you should reach more positive and negative muscle failure within the anaerobic energy system (under 90 seconds).

Pre-Exhaustion Training

If you prefer to do more than one set of exercise for a muscle group, you should try pre-exhaustion training. Pre-exhaustion training begins with a rotary (curved path) exercise to fatigue the target muscles (see figure 3.5a). Then you quickly perform a linear (straight path) exercise that brings in fresh assisting muscles to further fatigue the target muscles (see figure 3.5b). The first set should cause temporary muscle failure within 60 seconds (about 10 repetitions), and the follow-up set should

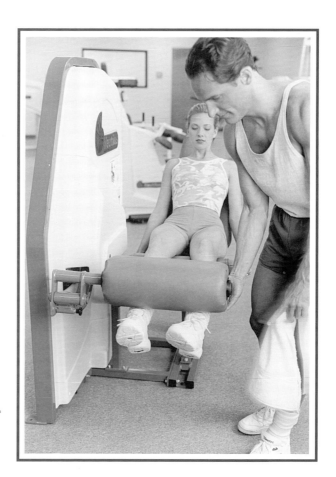

Fig. 3.4 With a training partner you can safely add a few more repetitions to achieve a high-intensity workout.

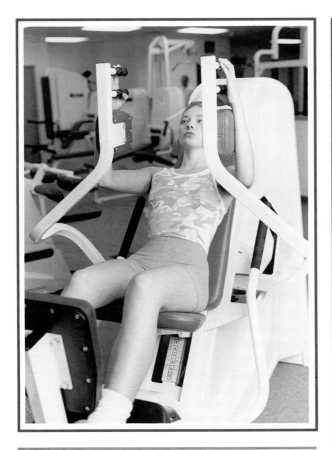

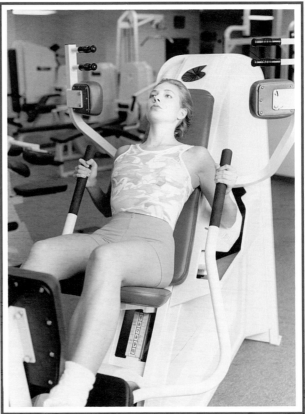

Fig. 3.5a A rotary exercise quickly exhausts the target muscles.

Fig. 3.5b A linear exercise uses assisting muscles that enable you to further fatigue the target muscles following the rotary exercise.

cause a temporary muscle failure within 30 seconds (about 5 repetitions). The successive exercises should give you two levels of muscle failure within the anaerobic energy system.

For example, when you perform two sets of bench presses with the same resistance, you activate the same pectoralis major muscle fibers twice. This increases the exercise duration but does not necessarily increase the exercise intensity. That is, you work the same muscle fibers more, rather than work more muscle fibers.

Instead, perform a set of arm crosses followed immediately by a set of decline presses on the Nautilus double chest machine. The arm cross is a rotary movement that targets the pectoralis major. When the pectoralis major reaches temporary muscle failure, you can no longer continue this exercise. But if you immediately perform the decline press, you can further fatigue the pectoralis major. The decline press is a linear movement that targets the pectoralis major and the triceps. The different movement pattern activates different motor units, and assistance from fresh triceps allows the fatigued pectoralis major to work even harder. (See table 3.6 for several pairs of rotary and linear exercises that provide pre-exhaustion training for most of the major muscle groups.)

Negative Training

Because of muscle friction, you can lower more resistance than you can lift. So if you eliminate the lifting movements, you can perform the lowering movements with heavier weight loads. This greater overload on your muscle further stimulates strength development.

Negative training is more demanding than standard training and it causes two problems. First, using heavier weight loads than you can lift increases the risk of injury to your muscles and connective tissue. Because negative contractions are associated with tissue microtrauma and delayed onset muscle soreness, you must not overdo negative training. Second, having partners lift heavy weight loads into the desired starting positions may be both difficult and dangerous.

For these reasons, you should not do negative training with extra-heavy weight loads. Instead, try assisted training that emphasizes negative muscle contractions with your standard resistance during the post-failure repetitions.

Exceptions to the rule on negative training include chin-ups and bar-dips with body weight. If you cannot lift your body weight, simply climb to the top position (full muscle contraction) and slowly lower yourself (negative muscle contraction) to the bottom position (full muscle stretch). Always have a partner present to help you in case you lose control of the lowering movement.

Table 3.6 Examples of pre-exhaustion exercises.		
Muscle group	**Rotary exercise**	**Linear exercise**
Quadriceps	Leg extension	Leg press
Hamstrings	Leg curl	Leg press
Deltoids	Lateral raise	Overhead press
Latissimus dorsi	Super pullover Behind-the-neck	Compound row Torso arm
Pectoralis major	10° chest 50° chest	Bench press Incline press
Biceps	Preacher curl	Chin-up
Triceps	Triceps extension	Bar-dip

Slow Training

Slow training is a form of high-intensity exercise that uses longer repetitions. The most common slow training procedure uses a 10-second lifting movement and a 4-second lowering movement. The slow and sustained lifting speed reduces momentum and increases muscle tension, which may enhance the training benefit. At 14 seconds a repetition, four to six repetitions are sufficient to fatigue the target muscles within the anaerobic energy system.

In spite of being tough and tedious to perform, slow training is a productive means for developing muscle strength (8). Subjects who did the slowest training gained more strength than those who used faster movement speeds (see table 3.3). Although the differences were not statistically significant, the trend favoring slow training appears to make this an effective high-intensity technique.

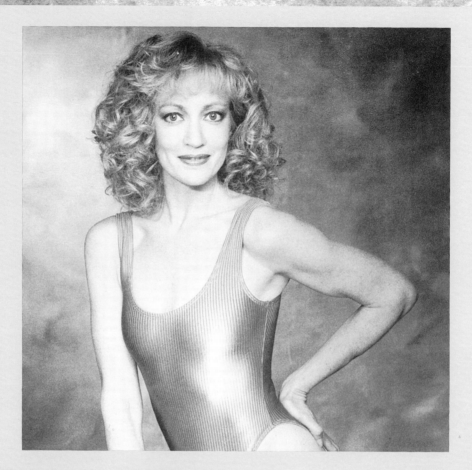

Candice Copeland is an internationally known choreographer and dance exercise specialist. Featured in eight videos (the latest being "Step 'n Low" and "Dynamic Stretch") and a frequent guest on television, she also writes and choreographs exercise videos for other fitness personalities. Candice has written two books, *Move* and *Thoroughly Fit*, and she has written for and appeared on the pages of such fitness magazines as *Shape*, *Self*, and *IDEA Today*.

Known best for her aerobics workouts, Candice also recognizes how important resistance training is to a well-rounded fitness routine. "Research and my own experience tell me that muscular strength is an important component of fitness that must be faithfully trained to maintain fitness," says Candice. "Each workout can take as little as 20 minutes. I carefully choose 8 to 10 exercises that challenge all the major muscle groups in the body, which is important for muscular balance. I've found that I don't have to live at the gym to train and maintain excellent gains in this important component of fitness—but I do have to be consistent in my commitment."

SUMMARY OF HIGH-INTENSITY TRAINING PROCEDURES

High-intensity training is an effective and efficient means for overcoming strength plateaus and enhancing muscle development. Rather than doing more exercise sets, high-intensity training makes each set more demanding.

High-intensity training may extend the exercise set through breakdown, assisted, or pre-exhaustion procedures, or it may extend the exercise repetition by decreasing the exercise speed as in slow training. Because all of the high-intensity techniques increase muscle stress, you should give yourself longer recovery and building periods after these workouts. For best results, do not perform high-intensity exercise sessions more than once or twice a week.

CHAPTER 4

Strength Training Equipment

Some people don't like technology. They prefer the simplicity of doing strength exercise without the bother of equipment—fancy or simple. They do sit-ups for their midsection, push-ups for their upper body, and knee bends for their lower body. But while these body weight exercises are beneficial up to a point, they don't permit progressive increases in training resistance. To better develop muscle strength, you must use enough resistance to fatigue the target muscles within the anaerobic energy system (about 8 to 12 repetitions in less than 90 seconds). As you become stronger and do more repetitions, you must add resistance to maintain a desirable repetition range.

THE DEVELOPMENT OF STRENGTH TRAINING EQUIPMENT

Because body weight exercises limit you to a single resistance, strength building enthusiasts have developed exercise equipment that has adjustable weight loads.

Early Strength Training Equipment

The basic barbell, introduced around the turn of the century, was one of the first adjustable strength training tools. As you gain strength, you add barbell plates to increase the weight load. Barbell training is unique because it is a simple, yet versatile, form of resistance exercise (see appendix A).

Resistance Exercise Machines

The next step in strength training equipment was the introduction of weight stack machines. The weight stacks, which always traveled vertically against gravity, were moved by means of attached handles or cables. These machines offered the convenience of changing resistance by merely inserting a pin and the safety feature of never being trapped under a heavy barbell.

In 1970, Nautilus developed a new line of resistance machines that attempted to imitate the muscle-joint function of the body. For example, the super pullover machine for the upper back (latissimus dorsi) muscles, incorporated several unique design features (see figure 4.1). The first functional design feature was a rotary movement arm that revolved around the shoulder joint axis to better isolate the latissimus dorsi and match human biomechanics.

The second functional design feature was direct resistance, with movement pads that touched the upper arms. The resistance force was applied directly to the upper arm where the latissimus dorsi attaches. Placing the resistance force against the upper arm rather than against the hand eliminated using the smaller forearm muscles and biceps, which usually tired before the larger latissimus dorsi.

The third functional design feature was variable resistance, accomplished by an oval-shaped cam that automatically changes the resistance force throughout the exercise movement. The cam proportionately increases the resistance in stronger segments of the movement range and proportionately decreases the resistance in weaker segments of the movement range. In this way, variable resistance tries to keep resistance force and muscle force well-matched throughout the exercise movement. This virtually

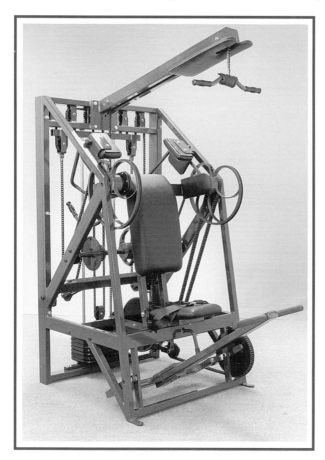

Fig. 4.1 Super pullover machine incorporates rotary movement, direct resistance, and variable resistance.

eliminates sticking points, or places in the movement range where the resistance is too heavy.

FEATURES AND ADVANTAGES OF FREE WEIGHT EXERCISE EQUIPMENT

Barbells and dumbbells are inexpensive tools that provide progressive resistance exercise for most of the major muscle groups. They take up little space and are easy to move from place to place. Free weights are versatile, simple to use, and almost indestructible; barbells and dumbbells have long been a popular choice for at-home strength training.

FEATURES AND ADVANTAGES OF RESISTANCE EXERCISE MACHINES

Resistance machines are designed to make strength exercise more efficient, safe, and productive.

Safety and Convenience Factors

Nautilus machines make each repetition more productive because they do a better job of isolating the target muscle and of matching resistance force to your potential muscle force. And by providing a supportive exercise structure, Nautilus machines keep you in a stable position that increases your movement range and stretches the muscles, reducing the risk of injury. The weight stack feature prevents the possibility of being trapped under a heavy barbell. It also eliminates the risk and bother of loading and unloading barbell plates because the resistance is easily changed by moving a pin. Another important safety feature is that resistance machines provide a specific movement path to keep the joint action on track throughout each exercise set. These features make resistance machines the preferred training mode for people who desire safe, simple, and brief exercise sessions.

Full-Range Exercise Factors

The Nautilus design features—rotary movement, direct resistance, and variable resistance—made the super pullover a safe, effective, and efficient machine for strengthening the latissimus dorsi. Nautilus later developed similar machines that targeted the other major muscle groups, while providing nine strength training factors known collectively as *full-range exercise.* Full-range exercise means that each training repetition is as productive as possible for stimulating strength development. This is accomplished through positive work, negative work, rotary movement, direct resistance, variable resistance, balanced resistance, resistance in full contraction, resistance in full stretch, and unrestricted movement speed. Table 4.1 shows how various types of resistance equipment address these nine factors of full-range strength training, which are discussed below.

Positive Work

Positive work refers to resistance during positive (concentric) muscle contractions, which is the lifting phase of the exercise. Strength training that uses static (isometric) muscle contractions runs a high risk of cardiovascular problems due to increased blood pressure. Strength training that uses only negative (eccentric) muscle contractions with heavier than normal resistance runs a high risk of muscular injury. Full-range exercise begins with positive work (see figure 4.2).

Negative Work

Negative work refers to resistance during negative (eccentric) muscle contractions, which is the lowering phase of the exercise. Because eccentric contractions cause more tissue microtrauma, negative work increases the strength-building stimulus. Remember that the same muscle lifts (positive contraction) and lowers (negative contraction) the resistance. Like positive work, negative work is an essential component of full-range exercise (see figure 4.3).

Rotary Movement

Every muscle contracts in a linear movement. But the bone attached to the contracting muscle is pulled in a rotary, or curved, movement. Con-

Table 4.1
How various types of resistance equipment address full-range exercise.

	Typical isokinetic equipment	Free weights	Typical weight stack machines	Nautilus machines
Positive work	All exercises	All exercises	All exercises	All exercises
Negative work	No exercises	All exercises	All exercises	All exercises
Rotary movement	All major muscle groups	Most major muscle groups	Most major muscle groups	All major muscle groups
Direct resistance	All major muscle groups	Some major muscle groups	Most major muscle groups	All major muscle groups
Variable resistance	All exercises	No exercises	Some exercises	All exercises
Balanced resistance	Not applicable	All exercises	Some exercises	All exercises
Resistance in full contraction	No exercises	Most exercises	All exercises	All exercises
Resistance in full stretch	No exercises	Most exercises	Most exercises	All exercises
Unrestricted movement speed	No exercises	All exercises	All exercises	All exercises

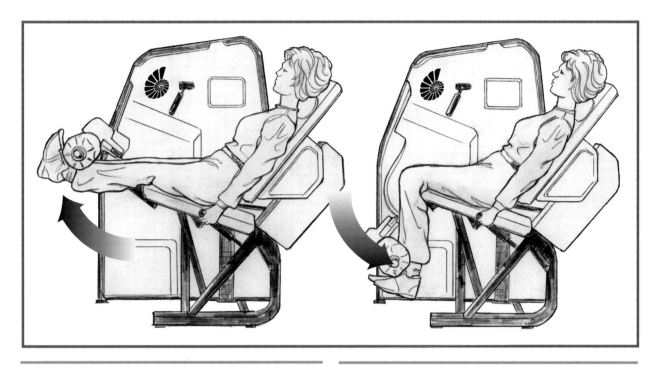

Fig. 4.2 Positive-work phase of leg extension exercise (quadriceps concentric contraction).

Fig. 4.3 Negative-work phase of leg extension exercise (quadriceps eccentric contraction).

sequently, to isolate a muscle, you must do rotary exercises (see figure 4.4). For example, the leg extension is a rotary exercise that isolates the quadriceps. The leg curl is a rotary exercise that isolates the hamstrings. In contrast, the leg press is a linear exercise that involves both the quadriceps and hamstrings. It is an excellent strength-building exercise that should be included in your overall training program, but it does not isolate a specific muscle group. Full-range training should include rotary movements that target each major muscle group.

Direct Resistance

To isolate a muscle most effectively, the resistance must be applied directly to the body part attached to that muscle. For example, to best isolate the deltoids, the re-

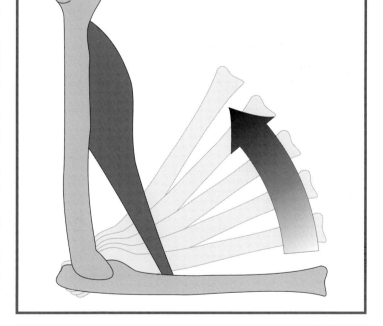

Fig. 4.4 Every muscle contracts in a straight line which pulls the attached bone in a rotary movement.

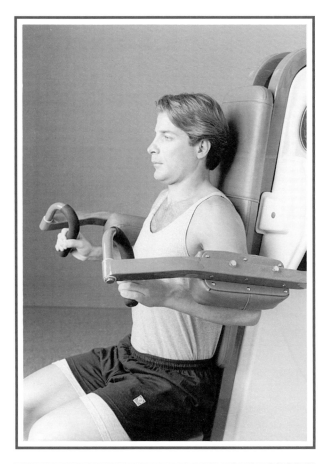

Fig. 4.5 Direct resistance applies resistance force directly to the target muscle.

sistance should be applied to the upper arm where the deltoids attach. This is why the lateral raise machine places the resistance pads directly against the upper arms (see figure 4.5). In contrast, the shoulder press applies the resistance to the hands, involving muscles in the forearms and upper arms, as well as the deltoids. Working with rotary movement, direct resistance enables you to effectively isolate the target muscle, making it an important component of full-range exercise.

Variable Resistance

Because of leverage factors, your muscle force is higher in some positions and lower in other positions. As a result, constant resistance exercise gives enough resistance in some parts of the movement range, but not enough resistance in other parts of the movement range. For example, in a leg press exercise you can apply 2.5 times more force in the last part than in the first part of the movement. To accommodate this large strength variation, the leg press machine uses a cam to automatically change the resistance force. The oval-shaped cam (figure 4.6) creates a counter-leverage system that provides proportionately less resistance in weaker segments of the movement range and proportionately more resistance in stronger segments of the movement range.

Because every muscle-joint action has a unique strength curve, every Nautilus machine has a specifically designed cam to automatically vary the resistance force throughout the exercise range. Variable resistance is an essential factor in full-range exercise.

Balanced Resistance

All exercise machines have moving parts that add and subtract resistance force, depending on the position of the movement arms. Well-designed machines are constructed with counterbalances to eliminate undesirable variations in the resistance force (see figure 4.7). The counterbalances cancel out the weight of the movement arms, so that the only resistance changes are those produced by the cam. Balanced resistance helps deliver the resistance force you want throughout your exercise movement.

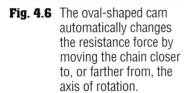

Fig. 4.6 The oval-shaped cam automatically changes the resistance force by moving the chain closer to, or farther from, the axis of rotation.

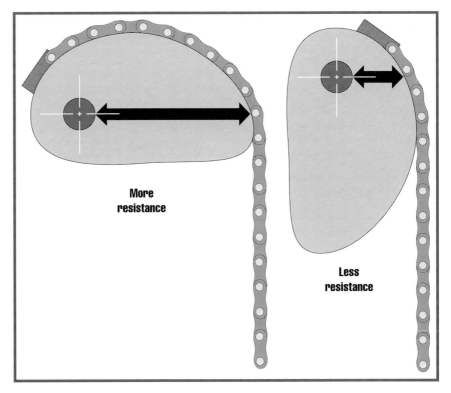

Resistance in Full Contraction

When you move a barbell outside the vertical plane, as some free weight exercises require, there may be no opposing resistance when your muscles are fully contracted. For example, when you perform dumbbell preacher bench curls the muscular effort drops off once your arms cross the vertical plane. At this point in the movement, gravity works for you, rather than against you, so there is no effective resistance when your biceps are fully contracted.

The Nautilus preacher curl machine eliminates this problem by using a vertical weight stack that always travels directly against the force of gravity (see figure 4.8). The movement arms are attached to the weight stack by means of a cam-chain or cam-belt arrangement that provides effective resistance throughout the entire movement range, even when your biceps are fully contracted. Because isokinetic machines provide resistance only when moving, they do not offer resistance in the fully contracted position. Resistance in full contraction is a necessary component of full-range exercise.

Resistance in Full Stretch

Full-range exercise requires that the target muscles work against appropriate resistance in every part of the movement range, including the position of full muscle stretch. Due to the interference of the bar itself, some barbell exercises do not allow resistance in the fully stretched position. The standing curl and bench press are examples of this problem. Well-designed machines have movement arms that provide variable re-

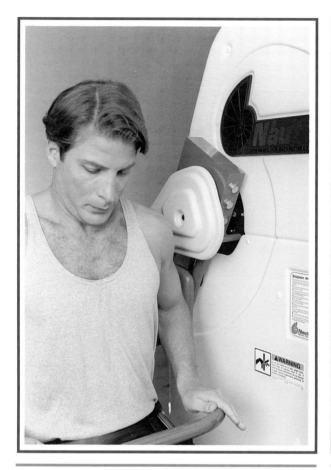

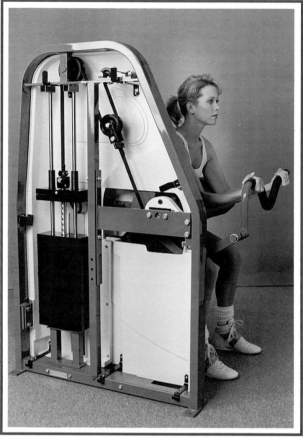

Fig. 4.7 Balanced resistance is accomplished by counterbalances to the movement arms.

Fig. 4.8 Weight stack moves directly against gravity regardless of the machine movement arm position.

sistance throughout the normal range of joint action, including the position of full muscle stretch (see figure 4.9).

Unrestricted Movement Speed

As presented in chapter 3, isometric exercise has no movement, while isokinetic exercise has a fixed movement speed. Nautilus machines provide a form of isotonic exercise that features both variable resistance and variable movement speed. Although fast training speeds are not advised because of inertia and momentum, no set speed for performing strength exercise exists. In fact, standard training involves two different movement speeds on every repetition. You should lift the weight load in two seconds and lower it in four seconds. By using these two movement speeds, you challenge the target muscles during both the weaker positive contraction (lifting phase) and the stronger negative contraction (lowering phase).

Prestretching

An advanced factor of full-range exercise, known as prestretching, is a controlled rebounding action between the end of one repetition and the start of the next. Although Nautilus once listed prestretching as the tenth

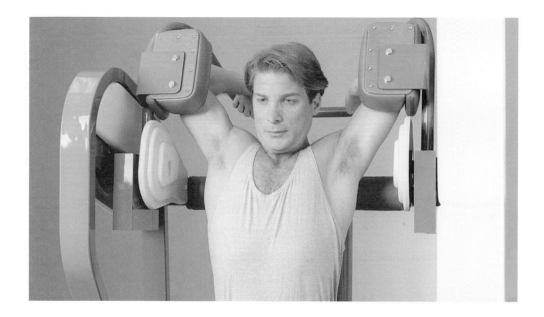

Fig. 4.9 Machine movement arms are designed to provide resistance throughout the exercise movement, including the position of full muscle stretch.

full-range exercise factor, recent research has shown that prestretching should only be attempted by highly-conditioned individuals. We therefore recommend it only for advanced exercisers and no longer include it in the basic list. For more information on prestretching, see chapter 13.

SUMMARY

Free weights provide a simple and effective means for doing progressive resistance exercise. You can use barbells and dumbbells for a variety of exercises. They take up little space and are almost maintenance-free, but require careful instruction and safety awareness.

Early weight stack machines increased exercise efficiency by eliminating the need to change barbell plates. They also increased training safety by preventing the possibility of being trapped under a heavy barbell.

Nautilus machines were designed to offer full-range strength training, including nine exercise components. The most important of these are rotary movement, direct resistance, and variable resistance. Rotary movement permits you to isolate the target muscle better than linear movement. Direct resistance is application of the resistance force to the body part controlled by the target muscle. Variable resistance provides a closer matching of muscle force and resistance force throughout the movement range. The other components of full-range strength training include positive work, negative work, balanced resistance, resistance in full contraction, resistance in full stretch, and unrestricted movement speed.

CHAPTER 5

Strength Training Exercises

Now you're ready to learn specific strength training exercises. Your job is to perform each exercise properly to develop the most strength. The exercises are grouped under the following categories based on the muscles addressed:

1. Leg exercises
2. Chest exercises
3. Upper back exercises
4. Shoulder exercises
5. Arm exercises
6. Midsection exercises
7. Neck exercises

Photographs of the beginning and ending positions accompany each exercise description. Nautilus equipment is featured because these machines are uniquely designed to provide all nine factors of full-range strength training, as discussed in chapter 4. (For those occasions when you do not have access to the equipment shown, refer to appendix A for free weight alternatives.)

BEFORE YOU BEGIN

Before you begin exercising, you should determine how each exercise fits into your overall training program. You must also be comfortable with your equipment and confident in your exercise technique. To give you a complete overview, be sure to read through both this chapter and the next before beginning your strength training.

Pre-Performance Checkpoints

Before starting your exercise set, you should check these key factors related to your positioning and performance:

1. Make sure you have placed the desired resistance on the weight stack.

   - See that the selector pin is inserted properly.
   - Add or remove saddle weights (2.5 lb., 5.0 lb., 7.5 lb.) as necessary to establish correct weight load.

2. Double-check your seat position to make sure that your joint axis of rotation is in line with the machine axis of rotation (rotary exercises) or set for a full range of joint movement (linear exercises). When you are properly positioned, the cam will correctly change the resistance to match your target muscle's strength throughout the exercise movement.

3. If seat belts are provided, be sure to fasten them snugly around your waist (super pullover, abdominal, torso arm, seated dip, and overhead press machines) or legs (low back and lower abdominal machines). Seat belts serve as anchors that help you maintain proper body alignment as you exercise.

4. Sit with proper posture and good back support. Your head should be in a neutral (upright) position on most machines.

5. If using free weights, make sure that the benches are stable, the racks are solid, and the plate collars are securely fastened.

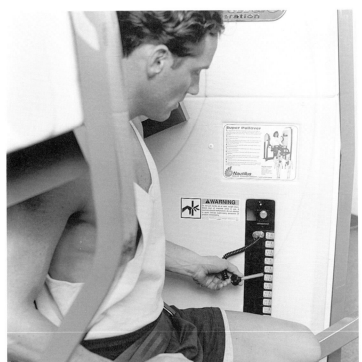

a

Select the weight load.

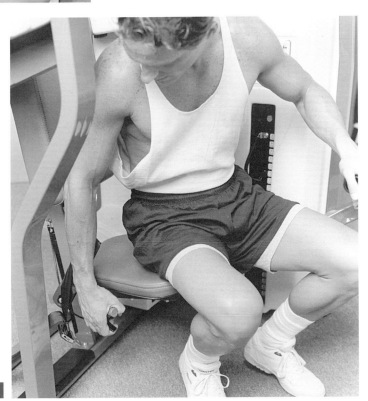

b

Adjust the seat.

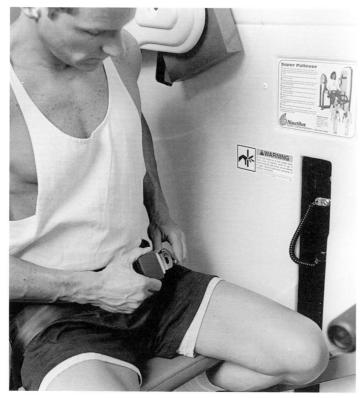

Secure the seatbelt.

Exercise Performance

When you perform your strength exercises, observe the following points to maximize muscle development and minimize injury risk:

- Perform each exercise slowly, about two seconds lifting and four seconds lowering. This standard six-second training procedure has consistently produced excellent results. The lowering phase is slower than the lifting phase to make the stronger negative (eccentric) muscle contractions more challenging.

- Perform each exercise through a full movement range. This is necessary for comprehensive muscle conditioning from the fully stretched to the fully contracted positions.

- Perform one set of each exercise. Single-set training is an effective and efficient means for increasing muscle strength and size.

- Use a weight load that fatigues the target muscles within 8 to 12 repetitions to emphasize the anaerobic energy system (about 50 to 70 seconds) and to develop more strength.

- Increase the weight load by 5 percent when 12 repetitions can be completed. Gradual training progression is the key to continued strength improvement with minimum risk of injuries.
- Breathe continuously throughout every repetition, exhaling while lifting and inhaling while lowering. This breathing pattern should reduce the chance of an excessive blood pressure response, while enhancing your exercise performance.
- Never compromise proper form for additional repetitions. Use proper technique to make sure that you are training the target muscles productively and safely.

Exercises for the larger muscle groups will be described first, then the exercises for the smaller muscle groups. This way, you will work with heavier weight loads when you are fresh and lighter weight loads when you are fatigued. This does not mean that the smaller muscles are less important than the larger muscles. But it is physiologically and psychologically better to perform higher-energy exercises before lower-energy exercises.

LEG EXERCISES

The following exercises address the largest and most-used muscles in the body. These are the quadriceps, hamstrings, gluteals, hip abductors, hip adductors, gastrocnemius, and soleus.

Hip and Back

Joint Action

Hip extension and trunk extension

Prime Mover Muscles

Hamstrings, gluteals, erector spinae

Movement Path

Rotary

Exercise Technique

- Pull brake lever and position the movement pad vertically.
- Lie on back with legs over the movement pad and hip joint in line with machine axis of rotation (red dot).
- Grip handles lightly.
- Extend legs and press movement pad downward to full muscle contraction.
- Return slowly to starting position and repeat.
- Grasp movement pad handle, pull brake lever, push movement pad away, and exit machine.

Technique Tips

- Keep head and shoulders on bench.
- Maintain snug belt to keep hips on bench.
- Extend hips within a comfortable range of movement.
- After a few repetitions pull movement pad handle backward for greater range of motion.

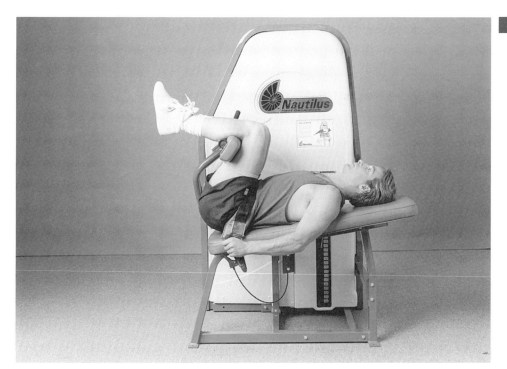

a

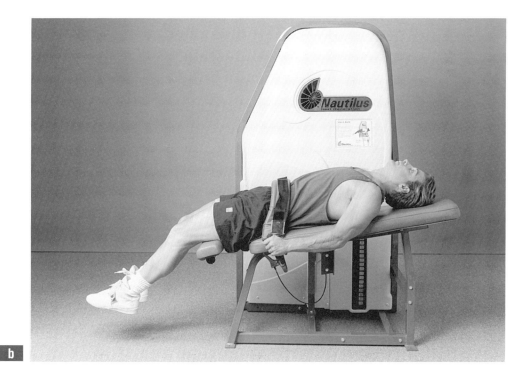

b

Leg Extension

Joint Action

Knee extension

Prime Mover Muscles

Quadriceps

Movement Path

Rotary

Exercise Technique

- Sit on seat and place legs behind adjustable movement pad.
- Align knees with machine axis of rotation (red dot).
- Push seat adjust lever to bring seat back against hips.
- Grip handles lightly.
- Lift movement pad until quadriceps are fully contracted.
- Return slowly to starting position and repeat.

Technique Tips

- Keep back against seat back.
- Maintain neutral head position.
- Keep ankles in neutral position (about 90°).

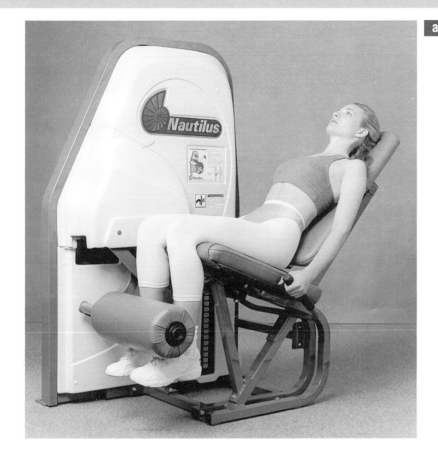

a

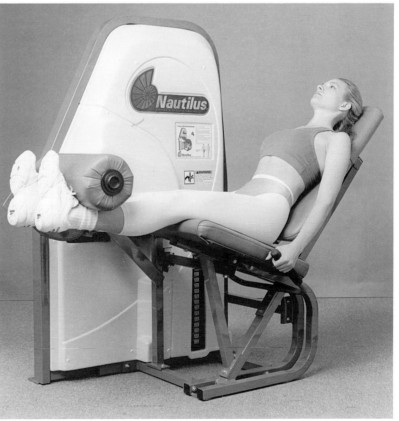

b

Seated Leg Curl

Joint Action

Knee flexion

Prime Mover Muscles

Hamstrings

Movement Path

Rotary

Exercise Technique

- Sit on seat, push leg entry handle forward, slide legs between adjustable movement pads, and return handle to resting position.
- Align knees with machine axis of rotation (red dot).
- Push seat adjust lever to bring seat back against hips.
- Grip handles lightly.
- Curl movement pad toward hips until hamstrings are fully contracted.
- Return slowly to starting position and repeat.

Technique Tips

- Keep back against seat back.
- Maintain neutral head position.
- Keep ankles in flexed position (toes pointed up).

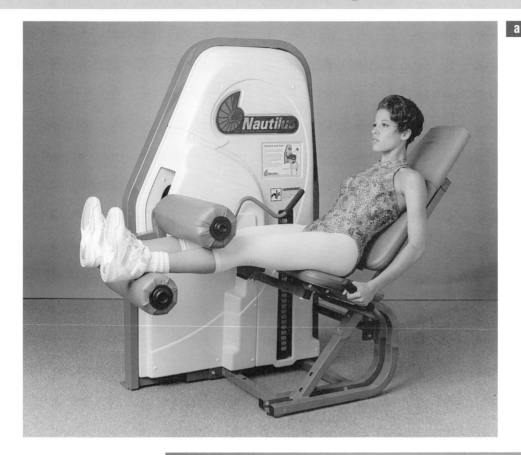

a

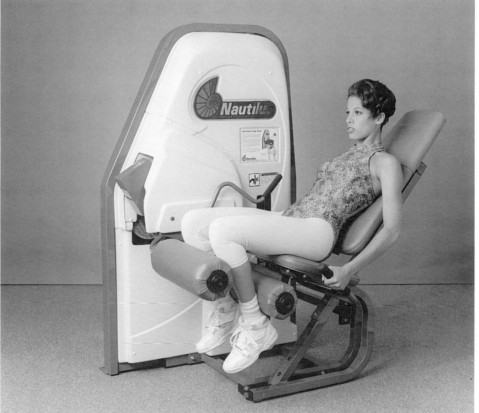

b

Prone Leg Curl

Joint Action

Knee flexion

Prime Mover Muscles

Hamstrings

Movement Path

Rotary

Exercise Technique

- Stand between bench seat and adjustable movement pad.
- Lie face down with legs straight and knees just off bench in line with machine axis of rotation (red dot).
- Grip handles lightly.
- Pull movement pad to hips by contracting hamstrings.
- Return slowly to starting position and repeat.

Technique Tips

- Keep chin on bench seat.
- Maintain hip support throughout exercise movement.
- Keep ankles in flexed position (toes pointed down).

Prone Leg Curl

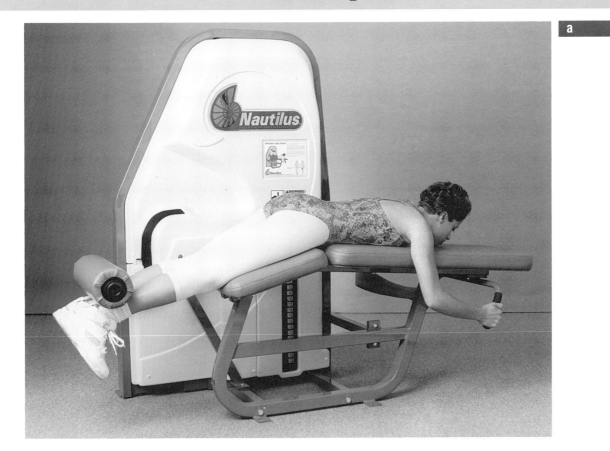

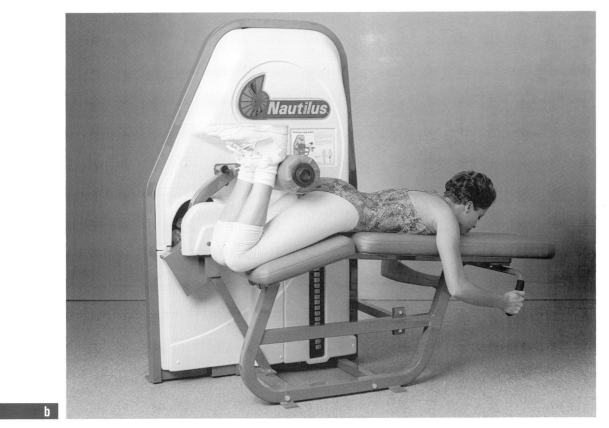

Leg Press

Joint Action

Hip extension and knee extension

Prime Mover Muscles

Hamstrings, gluteals, and quadriceps

Movement Path

Linear

Exercise Technique

- Sit with feet evenly placed on footpad, heels at bottom.
- Crank seat forward until knees are close to chest and directly behind feet.
- Grip handles lightly.
- Push footpad forward until knees are almost fully extended.
- Return slowly to starting position and repeat.

Technique Tips

- Keep back against seat back.
- Maintain neutral head position.
- Stop short of locking your knees.

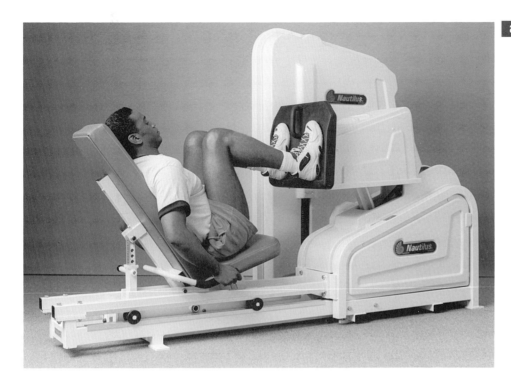

a

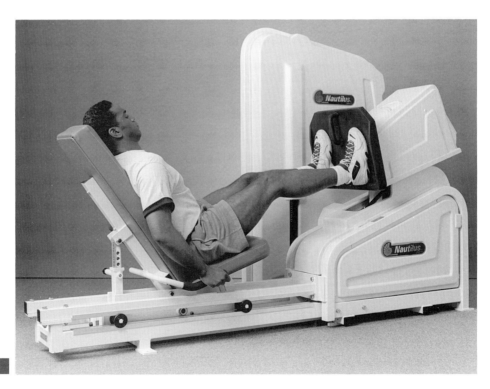

b

Hip Abductor

Joint Action

Hip abduction

Prime Mover Muscles

Hip abductors

Movement Path

Rotary

Exercise Technique

- Sit with hip joints aligned with machine axis of rotation.
- Place thighs inside movement pads.
- Grip handles lightly.
- Push movement pads apart as far as possible.
- Return slowly to starting position and repeat.

Technique Tips

- Keep back against seat back.
- Maintain neutral head position.
- Keep ankles in neutral position.

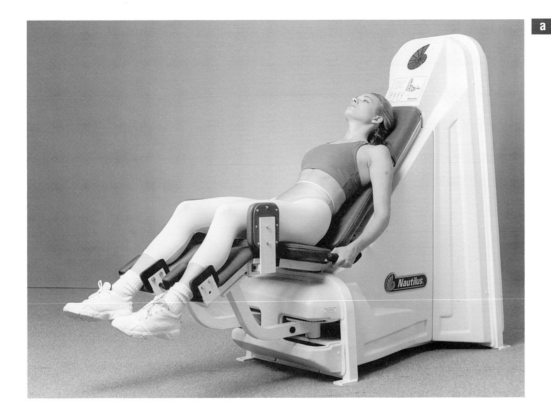

a

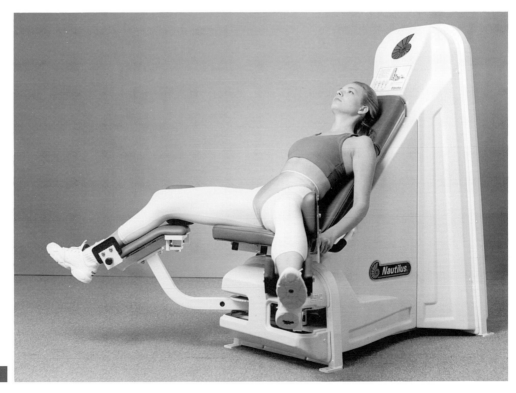

b

Hip Adductor

Joint Action

Hip adduction

Prime Mover Muscles

Hip adductors

Movement Path

Rotary

Exercise Technique

- Sit with hip joints aligned with machine axis of rotation.
- Place thighs outside movement pads.
- Grip handles lightly.
- Pull movement pads together until they make contact.
- Return slowly to starting position and repeat.

Technique Tips

- Keep back against seat back.
- Maintain neutral head position.
- Keep ankles in neutral position.

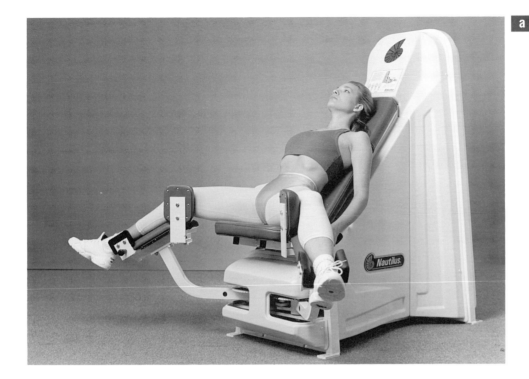

a

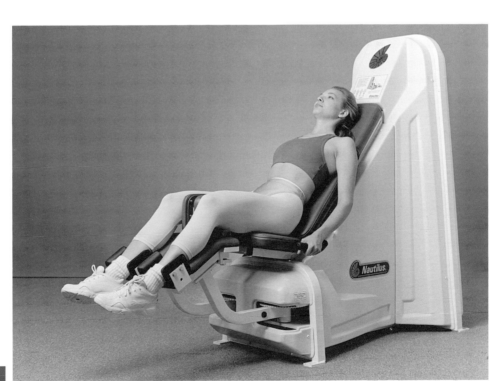

b

Seated Calf

Joint Action

Ankle extension

Prime Mover Muscles

Gastrocnemius and soleus

Movement Path

Rotary

Exercise Technique

- Sit with knees almost fully extended and feet evenly placed on footpad, heels at bottom.
- Grip handles lightly.
- Rotate footpad forward by extending ankles.
- Return slowly to starting position and repeat.

Technique Tips

- Keep back against seat back.
- Maintain neutral head position.

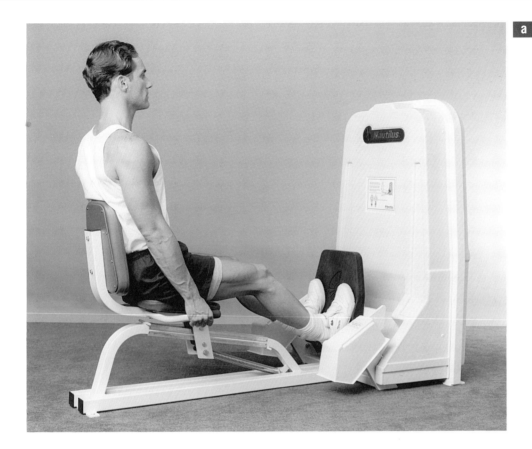

a

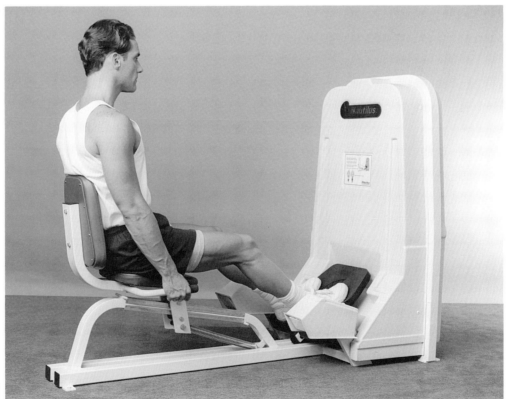

b

CHEST EXERCISES

The chest is one of the largest and most important muscle areas in the upper body. All of these exercises target the pectoralis major and anterior deltoid, and some include assisting muscles, such as the triceps.

Chest Cross

Joint Action

Shoulder horizontal flexion

Prime Mover Muscles

Pectoralis major and anterior deltoid

Movement Path

Rotary

Exercise Technique

- Sit with shoulder joints aligned with machine axis of rotation (red dots).
- Place elbows against elbow pads and palms against handles.
- Move elbow pads together as close as possible.
- Return slowly to starting position and repeat.

Technique Tips

- Keep back against seat back.
- Maintain neutral head position.
- Lead movements with elbows.
- When positioned properly, upper arms move parallel to floor.

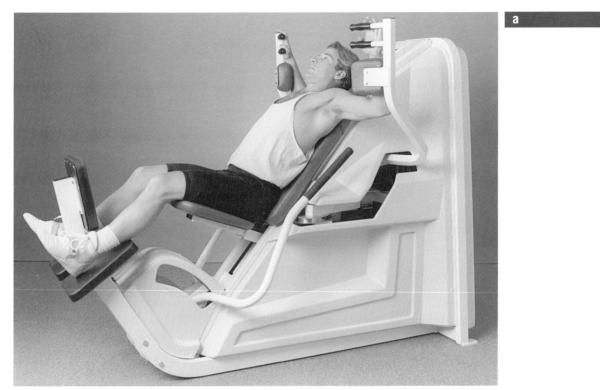

a

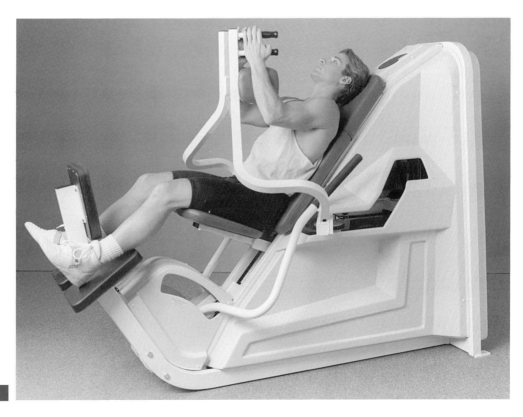

b

10° Chest

Joint Action

Shoulder horizontal flexion

Prime Mover Muscles

Pectoralis major and anterior deltoid

Movement Path

Rotary

Exercise Technique

- Lie with shoulder joints aligned with machine axis of rotation (red dots).
- Place upper arms under movement pads.
- Bring movement pads together until they make contact.
- Return slowly to starting position and repeat.

Technique Tips

- Keep head on bench.
- Keep feet on floor or footrest.
- When positioned properly, upper arms move perpendicular to floor.

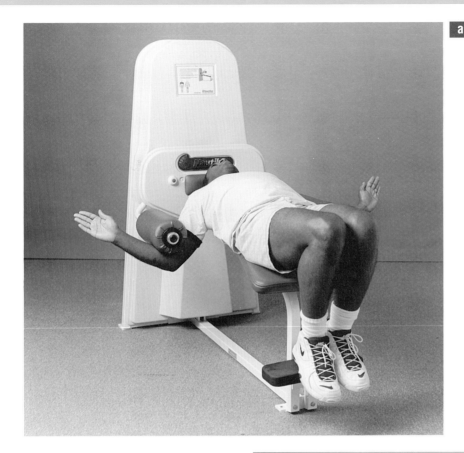

a

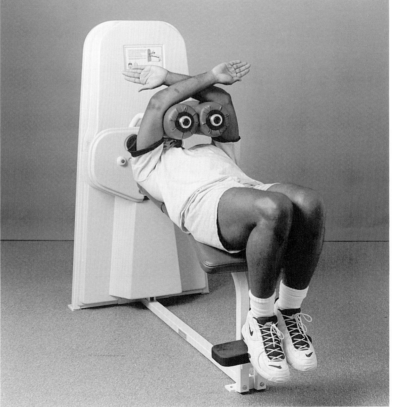

b

50° Chest

Joint Action

Shoulder horizontal flexion

Prime Mover Muscles

Pectoralis major and anterior deltoid

Movement Path

Rotary

Exercise Technique

- Sit with shoulder joints aligned with machine axis of rotation (red dots).
- Place upper arms under movement pads.
- Bring movement pads together until they make contact.
- Return slowly to starting position and repeat.

Technique Tips

- Keep head on headrest in horizontal position.
- When positioned properly, upper arms move perpendicular to floor.

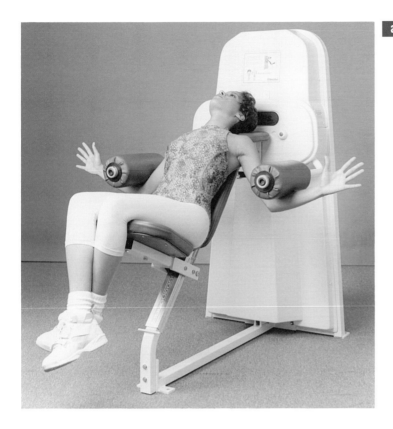

a

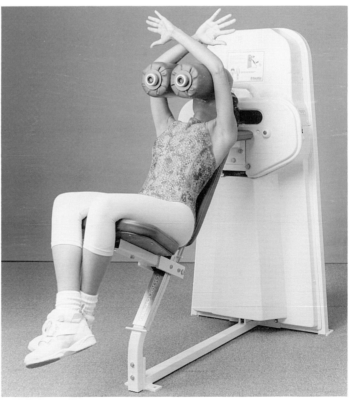

b

Bench Press

Joint Action

Shoulder horizontal flexion and elbow extension

Prime Mover Muscles

Pectoralis major, anterior deltoid, and triceps

Movement Path

Linear

Exercise Technique

- Lie with chest directly below handles.
- Grasp handles slightly wider than shoulders.
- Press handles upward until elbows are almost fully extended.
- Return slowly to starting position and repeat.

Technique Tips

- Keep head and hips on bench.
- Keep feet on floor or footrest.
- When positioned properly, upper arms finish perpendicular to floor.

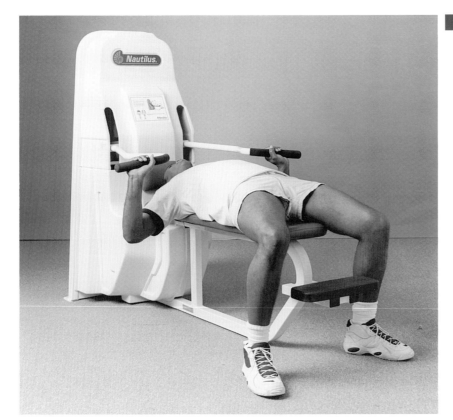

a

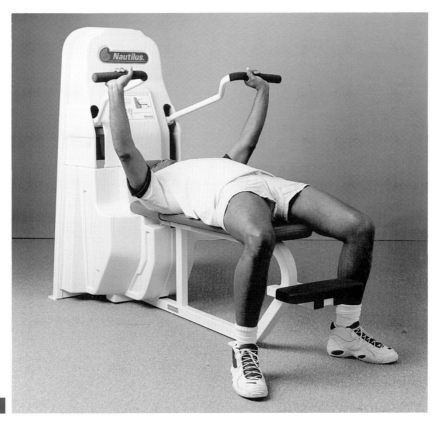

b

Decline Press

Joint Action

Shoulder horizontal flexion and elbow extension

Prime Mover Muscles

Pectoralis major, anterior deltoid, and triceps

Movement Path

Linear

Exercise Technique

- Sit with shoulders approximately even with handles.
- Place feet on footpad and press forward to position handles.
- Grasp handles and release footpad.
- Press handles forward until elbows are almost fully extended.
- Return slowly to starting position and repeat.
- After final repetition, place feet on footpad and press forward to reposition handles.

Technique Tips

- Maintain neutral head position.
- When positioned properly, upper arms finish approximately parallel to floor.

Decline Press

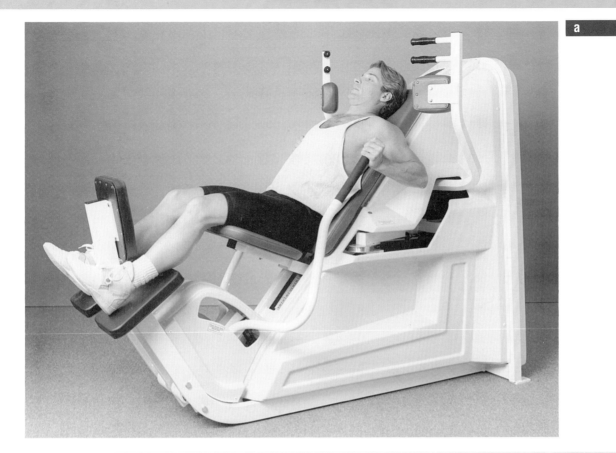

a

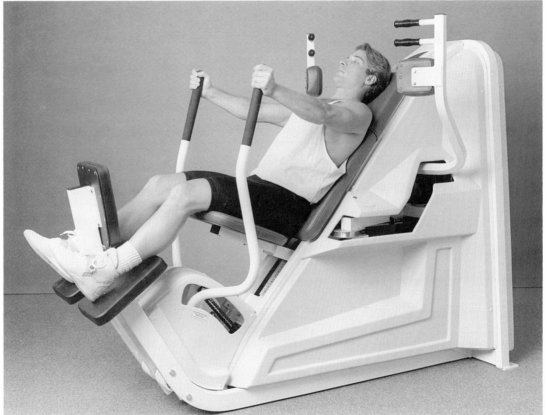

b

Incline Press

Joint Action

Shoulder horizontal flexion and elbow extension

Prime Mover Muscles

Pectoralis major, anterior deltoid, and triceps

Movement Path

Linear

Exercise Technique

- Sit with shoulders approximately even with handles.
- Press handles upward until elbows are almost fully extended.
- Return slowly to starting position and repeat.

Technique Tips

- Maintain neutral head position.
- When positioned properly, arms finish approximately perpendicular to floor.

Incline Press

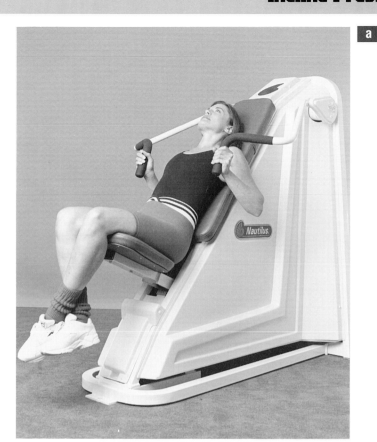

a

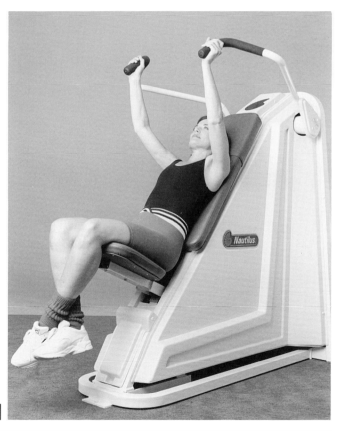

b

Seated Dip

Joint Action

Shoulder adduction and triceps extension

Prime Mover Muscles

Pectoralis major, latissimus dorsi, and triceps

Movement Path

Linear

Exercise Technique

- Sit with shoulders slightly above handles.
- Secure seat belt.
- Press handles downward until elbows are almost fully extended.
- Return slowly to starting position and repeat.

Technique Tips

- Body may lean slightly forward during exercise performance.
- Upper arms should be slightly below parallel to floor in top position.

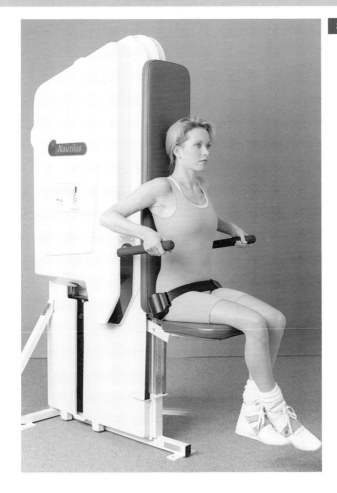

a

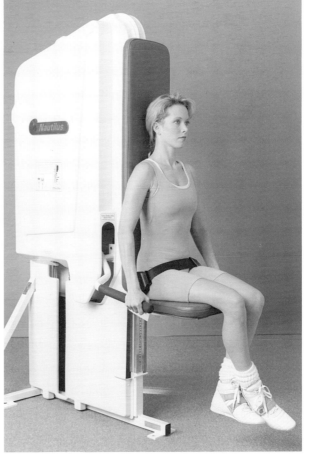

b

Although the upper back includes several muscle groups, the most prominent is the latissimus dorsi. The following upper back exercises focus on this large muscle group, as well as the teres major.

Super Pullover

Joint Action

Shoulder extension

Prime Mover Muscles

Latissimus dorsi and teres major

Movement Path

Rotary

Exercise Technique

- Squeeze seat adjust lever to sit with shoulders in line with machine axis of rotation (red dots).
- Secure seat belt and press foot lever to position movement pads.
- Place arms on movement pads, grip crossbar lightly, and stretch arms upward as far as comfortable.
- Pull arms downward until crossbar contacts mid-section.
- Return slowly to starting position and repeat.
- After final repetition, press foot lever and take arm off movement pads.

Technique Tips

- Curl trunk forward slightly during pulling movement to provide low back support against seat back.
- Lead movements with elbows.

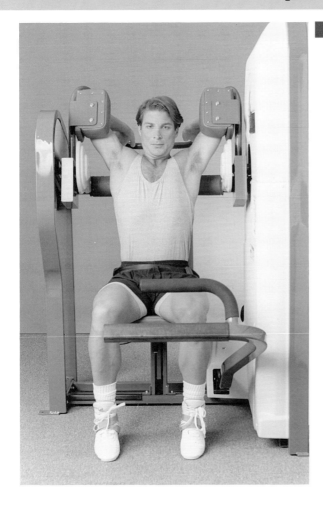

a

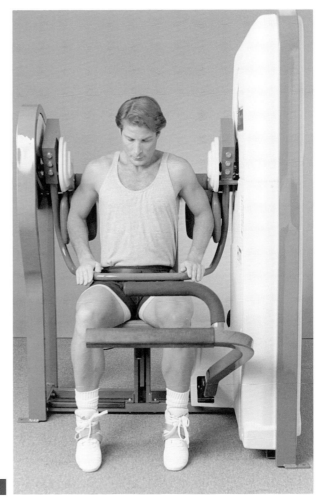

b

Rowing Back

Joint Action

Shoulder horizontal extension

Prime Mover Muscles

Posterior deltoid, latissimus dorsi, and teres major

Movement Path

Rotary

Exercise Technique

- Sit with shoulder joints aligned with machine axis of rotation (red dots).
- Place upper arms in movement pads, parallel to floor.
- Pull movement pads backward as far as possible.
- Return slowly to starting position and repeat.

Technique Tips

- Keep back against seat back.
- Maintain neutral head position.
- When positioned properly, upper arms move parallel to floor.

Rowing Back

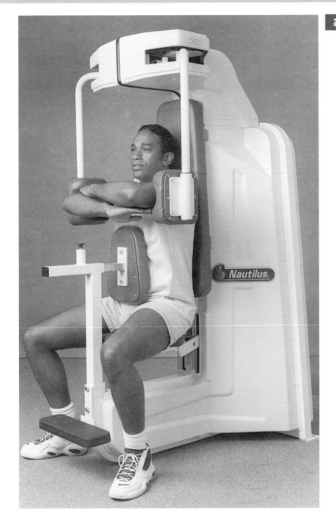

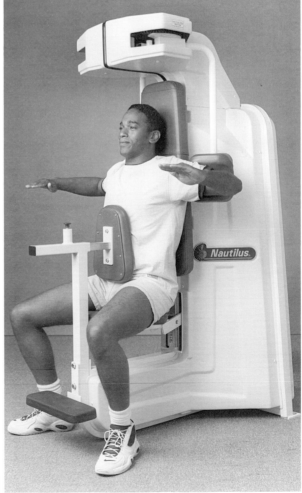

Behind-the-Neck

Joint Action

Shoulder adduction

Prime Mover Muscles

Latissimus dorsi, teres major, and pectoralis major

Movement Path

Rotary

Exercise Technique

- Sit with shoulder joints aligned with machine axis of rotation (red dots).
- Secure seat belt.
- Place upper arms inside movement pads.
- Pull movement pads downward until they make contact with body.
- Return slowly to starting position and repeat.

Technique Tips

- Keep back against seat back.
- Maintain neutral head position.
- When positioned properly, upper arms move perpendicular to floor.

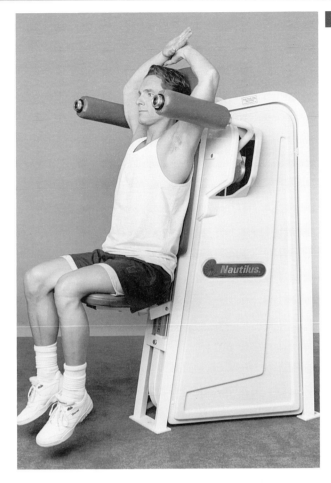

a

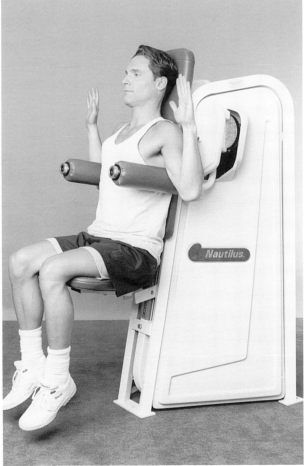

b

Torso Arm

Joint Action

Shoulder adduction and elbow flexion

Prime Mover Muscles

Latissimus dorsi, teres major, biceps

Movement Path

Linear

Exercise Technique

- Sit so that hands can just reach handles.
- Secure seat belt.
- Pull handles downward until hands are below shoulder.
- Return slowly to starting position and repeat.

Technique Tip

- Body may lean slightly forward during exercise performance.

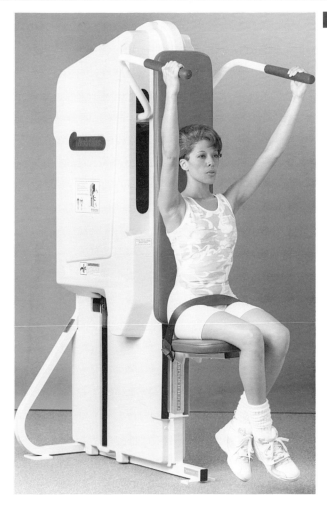

a

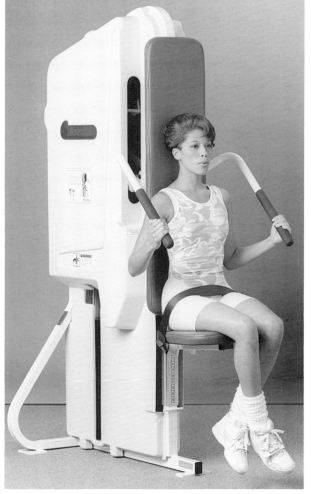

b

Compound Row

Joint Action

Shoulder extension and elbow flexion

Prime Mover Muscles

Latissimus dorsi, teres major, biceps

Movement Path

Linear

Exercise Technique

- Sit so that hands can just reach top of handles.
- Pull handles backward as far as possible.
- Return slowly to starting position and repeat.

Technique Tips

- Keep chest against restraining pad throughout exercise.
- Maintain neutral head position.
- Keep feet flat on floor.
- Grip may be either palms down or palms facing each other.

Compound Row

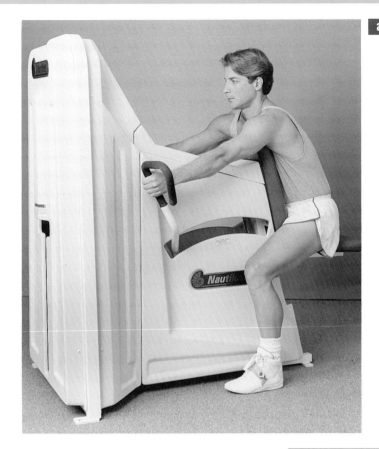

a

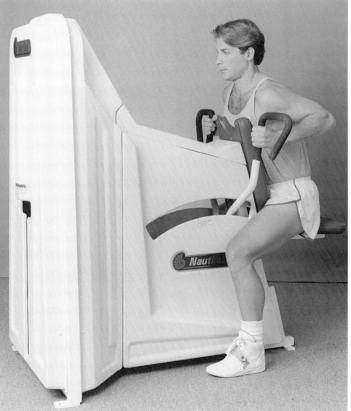

b

SHOULDER EXERCISES

The shoulder muscles include the larger deltoids and the smaller rotator cuff group. The following exercises are effective for strengthening these important shoulder joint muscles.

Lateral Raise

Joint Action

Shoulder abduction

Prime Mover Muscles

Deltoids

Movement Path

Rotary

Exercise Technique

- Squeeze seat adjust lever to sit with shoulders in line with machine axis of rotation (red dots).
- Place arms against sides inside the movement pads.
- Lift movement pads just above horizontal.
- Return slowly to starting position and repeat.

Technique Tips

- Keep back against seat back.
- Maintain neutral head position.
- Lead movements with elbows.

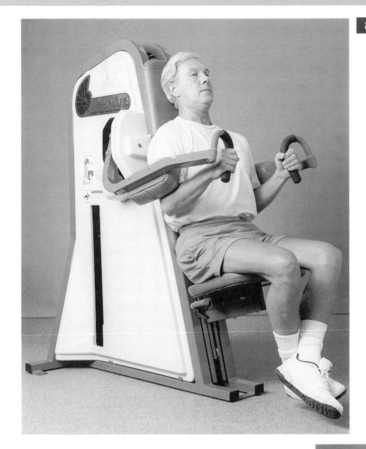

a

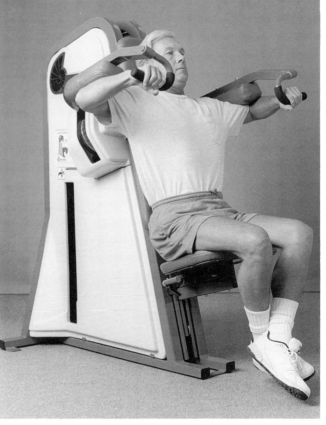

b

Overhead Press

Joint Action

Shoulder abduction and elbow extension

Prime Mover Muscles

Deltoids and triceps

Movement Path

Linear

Exercise Technique

- Sit with shoulders slightly lower than handles.
- Secure seat belt.
- Press handles upward until elbows are almost fully extended.
- Return slowly to starting position and repeat.

Technique Tips

- Keep back against seat back.
- Maintain neutral head position.
- Grip may be either palms facing each other or palms away.

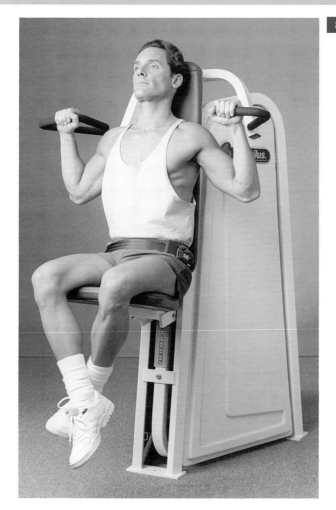

a

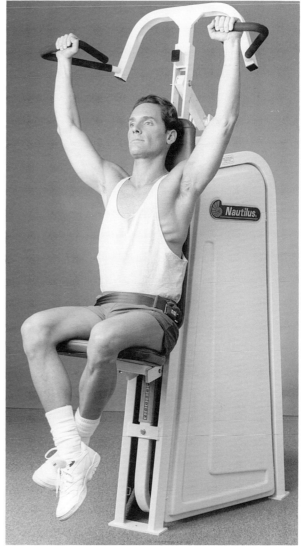

b

Rotary Shoulder

Joint Action

Shoulder inward rotation and shoulder outward rotation

Prime Mover Muscles

Shoulder inward rotators and shoulder outward rotators

Movement Path

Rotary

Exercise Technique

- Sit with shoulder joint in line with machine axis of rotation (red dots).
- Set selection lever for inward rotation.
- Place upper arm in cuff and grasp handle comfortably.
- Move handle forward as far as possible.
- Set selection lever for outward rotation.
- Place upper arm in cuff and grasp handle comfortably.
- Move handle backward as far as possible.
- Repeat procedure for other shoulder.

Technique Tips

- Keep back against seat back.
- Maintain neutral head position.

Rotary Shoulder

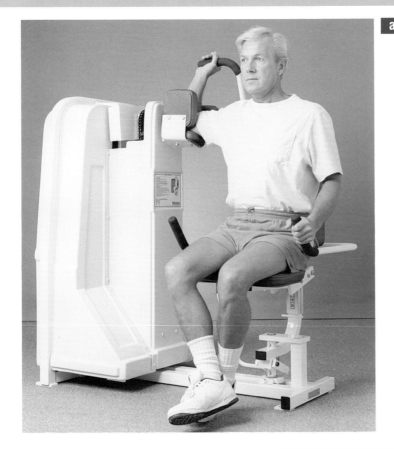

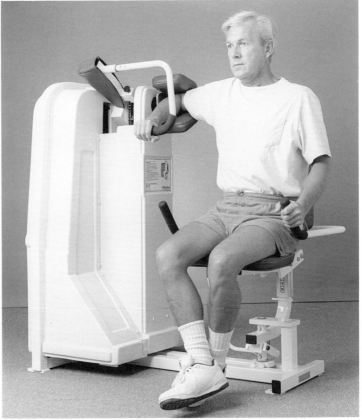

ARM EXERCISES

Although the biceps and triceps are the dominant muscles in the upper arm, the forearm muscles are also important. This section includes exercises for all of these muscle groups.

Preacher Curl

Joint Action

Elbow flexion

Prime Mover Muscles

Biceps

Movement Path

Rotary

Exercise Technique

- Squeeze seat adjust lever to sit with elbows in line with machine axis of rotation (red dots).
- Partially stand, grip movement bar loosely, and sit in properly aligned position.
- Curl movement bar upward as far as possible.
- Return slowly to starting position and repeat.
- After final repetition, partially stand and lower movement bar to resting position.

Technique Tips

- Maintain erect posture.
- Maintain neutral head position.
- It is not necessary to fully extend the elbows between repetitions.

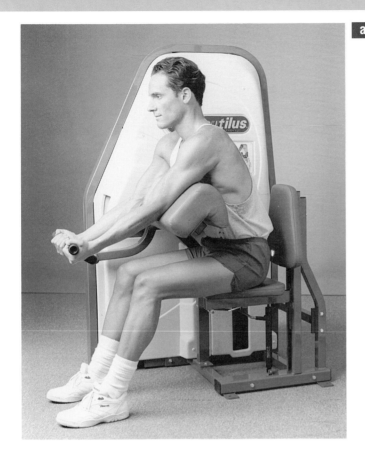

a

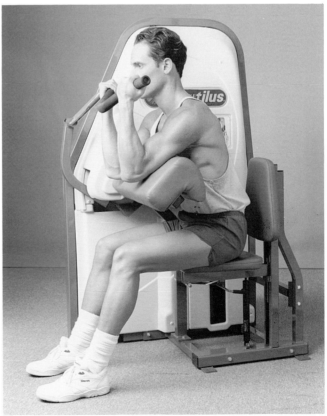

b

Triceps Extension

Joint Action

Elbow extension

Prime Mover Muscles

Triceps

Movement Path

Rotary

Exercise Technique

- Adjust back support and squeeze seat adjust lever to sit with elbows in line with machine axis of rotation (red dot).
- Place sides of hands on movement pads and begin with movement pads beside face.
- Extend arms downward until triceps are fully contracted.
- Return slowly to starting position and repeat.

Technique Tips

- Keep back against seat back.
- Maintain neutral head position.
- It is not necessary to fully flex the elbows between repetitions.

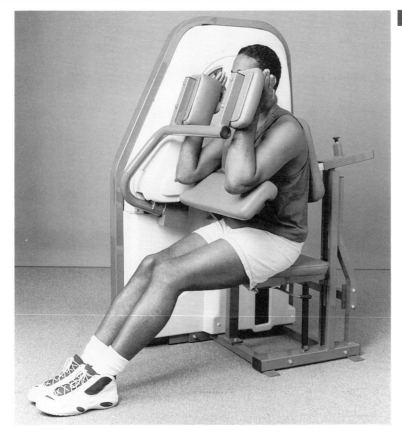

a

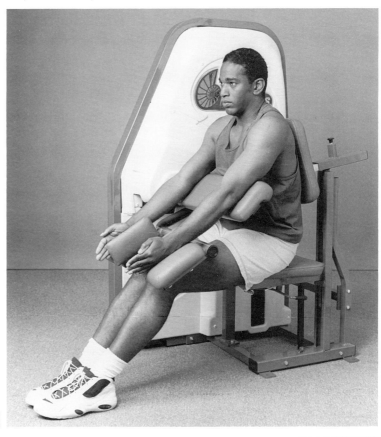

b

Super-Forearm

Joint Action

Wrist flexion, wrist extension, wrist inward rotation, wrist outward rotation

Prime Mover Muscles

Forearm flexors and forearm extensors

Movement Path

Rotary

Exercise Technique

- Sit with forearms approximately parallel to floor.
- Grasp appropriate handles and move in designated manner as illustrated on machine chart.

Technique Tips

- Maintain erect posture.
- Maintain neutral head position.

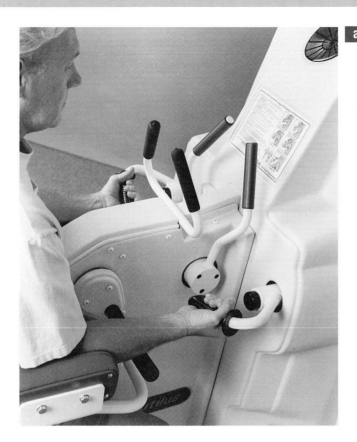

a

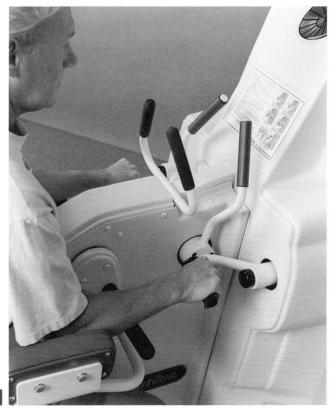

b

MIDSECTION EXERCISES

Midsection conditioning involves more than the abdominal muscles. In addition to the rectus abdominis, the erector spinae, internal obliques, external obliques, and hip flexor muscles all contribute to a strong midsection. This section includes exercises for each of these muscle groups.

Abdominal

Joint Action

Trunk flexion

Prime Mover Muscles

Rectus abdominis

Movement Path

Rotary

Exercise Technique

- Push the seat adjust lever to sit with navel in line with red dot.
- Anchor feet under adjustable foot pads.
- Place elbows on movement pads and grip handles lightly.
- Pull chest toward hips in crunch movement until abdominal muscles are fully contracted.
- Return slowly to starting position and repeat.

Technique Tips

- Keep upper back against seat back.
- Keep head neutral or slightly forward.

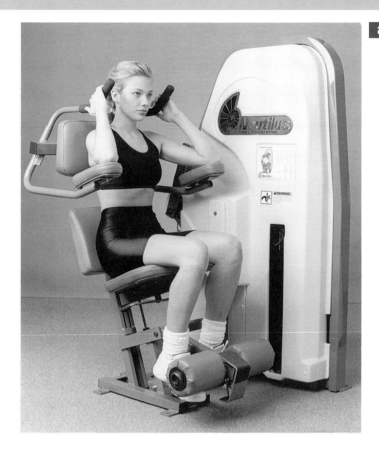

a

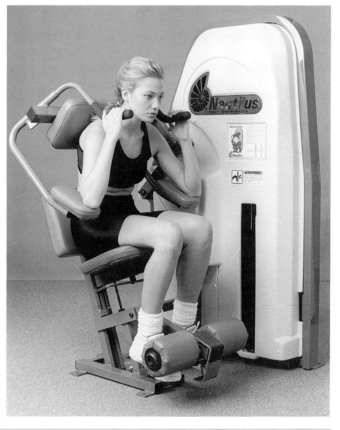

b

Low Back

Joint Action

Trunk extension

Prime Mover Muscles

Erector spinae

Movement Path

Rotary

Exercise Technique

- Push seat adjust lever to sit with navel in line with red dot.
- Position foot pad so knees are slightly higher than hips.
- Secure seat belts across shins and hips.
- Push movement pad backward until low back muscles are fully contracted.
- Return slowly to starting position and repeat.

Technique Tips

- Keep hips against seat back.
- Maintain neutral head position.

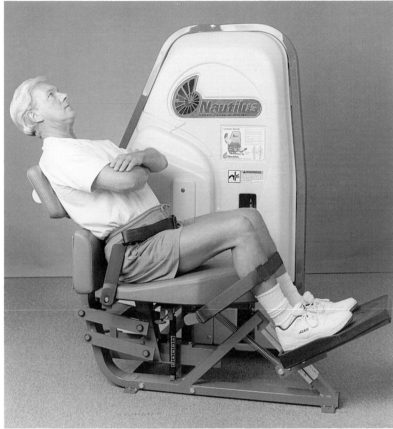

a

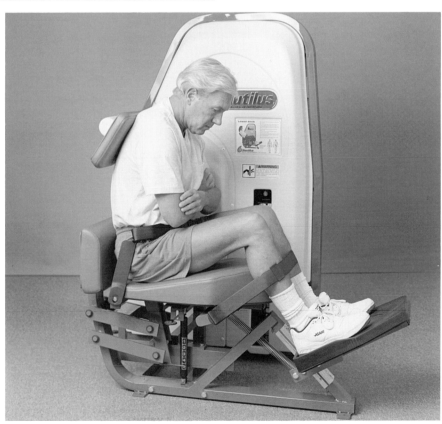

b

Rotary Torso

Joint Action

Trunk rotation

Prime Mover Muscles

External obliques and internal obliques

Movement Path

Rotary

Exercise Technique

- Sit with hips against seat ridge.
- Place arms behind arm pads.
- Turn torso clockwise until oblique muscles are fully contracted, return slowly, and repeat.
- Adjust seat position.
- Turn torso counterclockwise until oblique muscles are fully contracted, return slowly, and repeat.

Technique Tips

- Maintain erect posture.
- Maintain neutral head position.
- When hips are stabilized, the trunk has a relatively short rotation range.

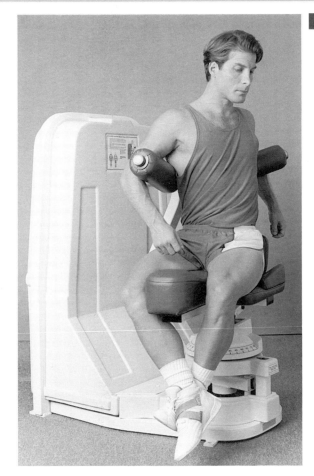

a

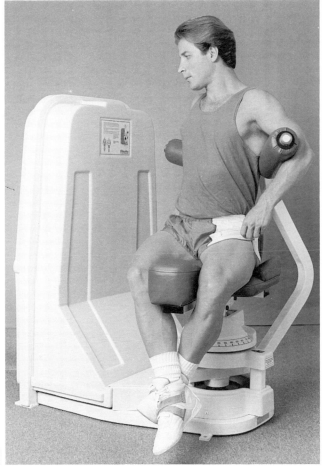

b

Lower Abdominal

Joint Action

Hip flexion

Prime Mover Muscles

Hip flexors and rectus abdominis

Movement Path

Rotary

Exercise Technique

- Lie with hip joints aligned with machine axis of rotation (red dot).
- Secure seat belt and grasp handles.
- Lift knees upward and backward as far as possible.
- Return slowly to starting position and repeat.

Technique Tips

- Keep back on bench.
- Keep head neutral or slightly forward.

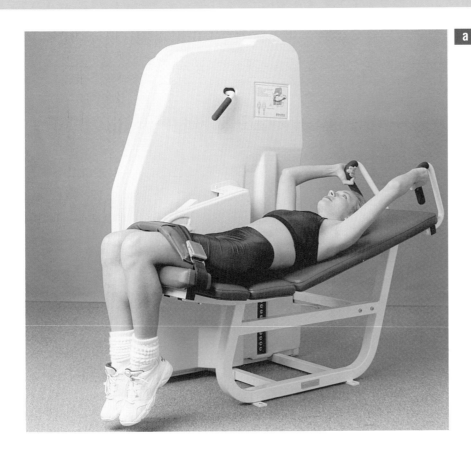

a

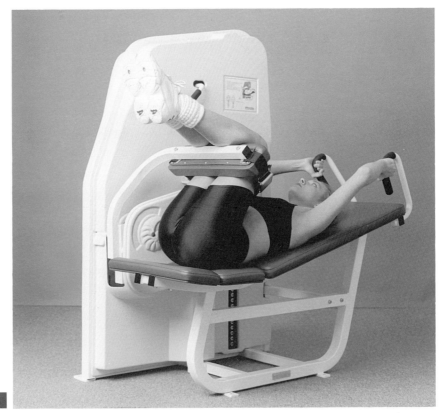

b

NECK EXERCISES

The neck is a vulnerable area of the body and should be included in every strength training program. The following exercises work on all of the neck muscles.

4-Way Neck

Joint Action

Neck flexion, neck extension, and neck lateral flexion

Prime Mover Muscles

Sternocleidomastoids, upper trapezius, and levator scapulae

Movement Path

Rotary

Exercise Technique

- Sit with face against movement pad. Grasp handles loosely. Push movement pad forward as far as possible (photos a and b). Return slowly to starting position and repeat.
- Sit with rear of head against movement pad. Grasp handles loosely. Push movement pad backward as far as possible (photos c and d). Return slowly to starting position and repeat.
- Sit with side of head against movement pad. Grasp handles loosely. Push movement pad sideward as far as possible (photos e and f). Return slowly to starting position and repeat.
- Sit with other side of head against movement pad. Grasp handles loosely. Push movement pad sideward as far as possible. Return slowly to starting position and repeat.

Technique Tips

- Maintain erect posture.
- Keep torso in contact with restraining pad.

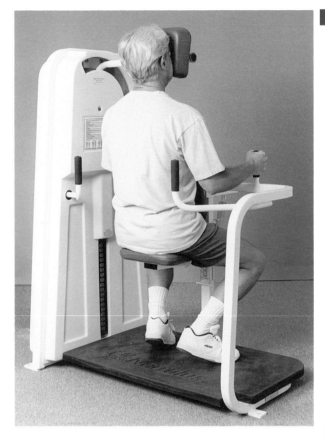

a

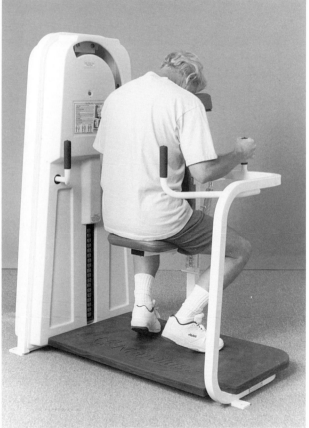

b

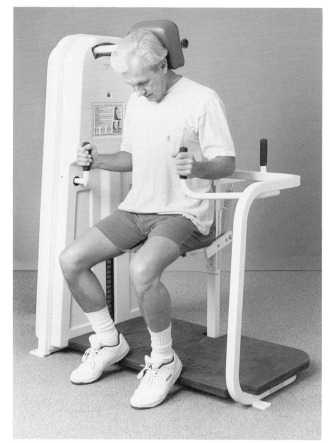

c

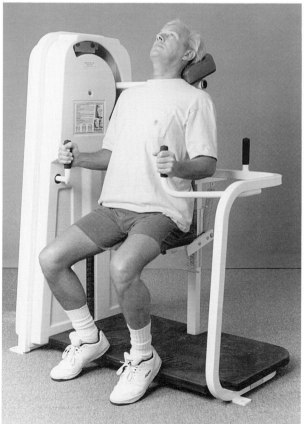

d

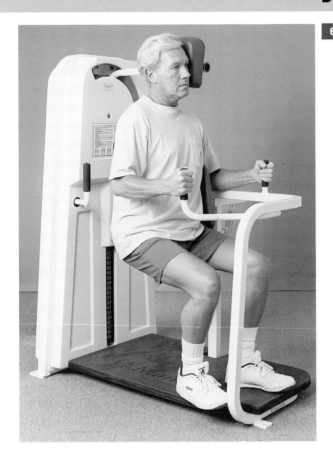

e

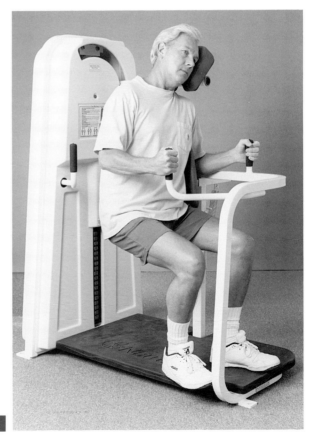

f

SUMMARY

Well-designed strength exercises facilitate safe, effective, and efficient training. To maximize strength development and minimize injury risk, follow these exercise performance guidelines:

- Select the desired resistance.
- Set the seat position for proper alignment.
- Use seat belts whenever they are provided.
- Sit with proper posture, good back support, and neutral head position.
- Train with a slow movement speed.
- Train with a full movement range.
- Use a weight load that fatigues the target muscles within 8 to 12 repetitions.
- Increase the weight load by 5 percent when you can complete 12 repetitions.
- Breathe continuously during every repetition.
- Never compromise proper form for additional repetitions.

Finally, do your best to perform each exercise in the way described. Deviations from the recommended training technique may reduce the effectiveness of the exercise and increase the risk of injury.

This chapter has taught you how to perform specific strength exercises; the following chapter will show you how to design a productive strength training program. Together, these chapters should enable you to have safe, effective, and efficient strength training experiences.

CHAPTER 6

Six-Month Strength Training Program

Now that you're familiar with the strength exercises, you need to know how to select and organize them into a systematic and successful training program.

It's best to begin with a few basic strength training exercises, then gradually increase the number of exercises as your muscles become better conditioned. This establishes a solid base of support in your major muscle groups and permits progressive strength development. You should also do different strength exercises as your muscles become accustomed to your standard training routine. This prevents boredom and enhances the training effect. Although your exercise facility may not have all of the equipment listed here, use this sample six-month training program as a guide for achieving better strength fitness, adapting the program to your needs and available equipment. This program is a highly effective and efficient means for muscular conditioning. Of course, you may repeat a month if you do not feel ready for the next training progression.

MONTH ONE

This is your first month of serious and sensible strength exercise, so you must begin slowly to maximize positive muscle responses and prevent overdoing it. If you stay with the recommended exercise program, you should make excellent progress without experiencing any training setbacks. This month of training will be described week-by-week.

Table 6.1
Muscles addressed by three Nautilus machines: Month one, week one.

Major muscle group	Machine
1. Quadriceps	Leg press
2. Hamstrings	Leg press
3. Hip adductors	X X X
4. Hip abductors	X X X
5. Pectoralis major	Decline press
6. Latissimus dorsi	Compound row
7. Deltoids	X X X
8. Biceps	Compound row
9. Triceps	Decline press
10. Low back	X X X
11. Abdominals	X X X
12. Neck	X X X

Month One, Week One

Begin with three basic exercises that address many of your key muscle areas. These are the leg press machine, the decline press machine, and the compound row machine (see program 6.1). These three machines use 6 out of 12 major muscle groups (see table 6.1).

Because all of these exercises are linear in nature, involving pushing or pulling in a straight line, they address more than one muscle group at the same time. By design, these exercises involve familiar movements that are important for daily activities and sport performance. The leg press strengthens both the quadriceps and hamstrings. The decline press strengthens the pectoralis major and triceps, and the

PROGRAM 6.1

Recommended program of strength exercise for the first week of training.

Exercise order	Training sets	Training repetitions	Training speed‡
1. Leg press*	1	8-12	2/4
2. Decline press*	1	8-12	2/4
3. Compound row*	1	8-12	2/4

* New exercises this week
‡Up and down in seconds

Table 6.2
Typical beginning weight loads for selected Nautilus machines by age and gender.

Age group	Leg press*	Decline press*	Compound row*
20-29			
Males	150.0	65.0	85.0
Females	100.0	40.0	55.0
30-39			
Males	137.5	60.0	80.0
Females	92.5	37.5	52.5
40-49			
Males	125.0	55.0	75.0
Females	85.0	35.0	50.0
50-59			
Males	112.5	50.0	70.0
Females	77.5	32.5	47.5
60-69			
Males	100.0	45.0	65.0
Females	70.0	30.0	45.0
70-79			
Males	87.5	40.0	60.0
Females	62.5	27.5	42.5

*Weight load in pounds

compound row stresses the latissimus dorsi and biceps. You should do one set of 8 to 12 repetitions with each exercise. When you can do 12 repetitions, increase your training resistance by about 5 percent. Table 6.2 gives typical starting weight loads for these exercises based on your age and gender. Your actual starting weight loads must be determined by personal trial, beginning with light resistance and adding weight until you are in the 8- to 12-repetition range. If you cannot complete 8 repetitions, reduce the resistance to prevent overstressing your muscles and joints.

Month One, Week Two

During the second week of training you may add two new exercises—the low back machine and the abdominal machine. Program 6.2 lists the recommended exercise order, and table 6.3 shows the major

PROGRAM 6.2

Recommended program of strength exercise for the second week of training.

Exercise order	Training sets	Training repetitions	Training speed‡
1. Leg press	1	8-12	2/4
2. Decline press	1	8-12	2/4
3. Compound row	1	8-12	2/4
4. Low back*	1	8-12	2/4
5. Abdominal*	1	8-12	2/4

*New exercises this week
‡Up and down in seconds

Table 6.3
Muscles addressed by five Nautilus machines: Month one, week two.

Major muscle group	Machine
1. Quadriceps	Leg press
2. Hamstrings	Leg press
3. Hip adductors	X X X
4. Hip abductors	X X X
5. Pectoralis major	Decline press
6. Latissimus dorsi	Compound row
7. Deltoids	X X X
8. Biceps	Compound row
9. Triceps	Decline press
10. Low back	Low back
11. Abdominals	Abdominal
12. Neck	X X X

Table 6.4
Typical beginning weight loads for selected Nautilus machines by age and gender.

Age group	Low back*	Abdominal*
20-29		
Males	70.0	70.0
Females	50.0	45.0
30-39		
Males	65.0	65.0
Females	47.5	42.5
40-49		
Males	60.0	60.0
Females	45.0	40.0
50-59		
Males	55.0	55.0
Females	42.5	37.5
60-69		
Males	50.0	50.0
Females	40.0	35.0
70-79		
Males	45.0	45.0
Females	37.5	32.5

*Weight load in pounds

muscle groups these five exercises address.

The low back and abdominal exercises are rotary in nature (moving in an arc around a rotational axis) and, as indicated by their names, target the low back and abdominal muscles. Perform one set of 8 to 12 repetitions with each exercise. When you can do 12 repetitions, increase your training resistance by about 5 percent. Table 6.4 lists typical starting weight loads for these exercises based on your age and gender.

Because low back problems and midsection weaknesses are quite common, begin these exercises with less than the standard starting weight loads. It is always better to begin too light and add resistance than to begin too heavy and risk injury.

Month One, Week Three

This is a good week to add two new leg exercises—the hip adductor machine and the hip abductor machine. The recommended machine order is listed in program 6.3 and the major muscle groups addressed by this program are noted in table 6.5.

The hip adductor machine works the inner thigh muscles, and the hip abductor machine targets the outer thigh muscles. Both are rotary exercises that strengthen the muscles responsible for lateral movement activities such as skating, skiing, tennis, and basketball.

Do one set of 8 to 12 repetitions of each exercise. When you can do 12 repetitions, increase your training resistance by about 5 percent. Table 6.6 lists typical starting weight loads for these new leg exercises based on your age and gender.

PROGRAM 6.3

Recommended program of strength exercise for the third week of training.

Exercise order	Training sets	Training repetitions	Training speed‡
1. Leg press	1	8-12	2/4
2. Hip adductor*	1	8-12	2/4
3. Hip abductor*	1	8-12	2/4
4. Decline press	1	8-12	2/4
5. Compound row	1	8-12	2/4
6. Low back	1	8-12	2/4
7. Abdominal	1	8-12	2/4

* New exercises this week
‡ Up and down in seconds

Table 6.5
Muscles addressed by seven Nautilus machines: Month one, week three.

Major muscle group	Machine
1. Quadriceps	Leg press
2. Hamstrings	Leg press
3. Hip adductors	Hip adductor
4. Hip abductors	Hip abductor
5. Pectoralis major	Decline press
6. Latissimus dorsi	Compound row
7. Deltoids	X X X
8. Biceps	Compound row
9. Triceps	Decline press
10. Low back	Low back
11. Abdominals	Abdominal
12. Neck	X X X

Table 6.6
Typical beginning weight loads for selected Nautilus machines by age and gender.

Age group	Hip abductor*	Hip adductor*
20-29		
Males	70.0	80.0
Females	45.0	55.0
30-39		
Males	65.0	75.0
Females	42.5	52.5
40-49		
Males	60.0	70.0
Females	40.0	50.0
50-59		
Males	55.0	65.0
Females	37.5	47.5
60-69		
Males	50.0	60.0
Females	35.0	45.0
70-79		
Males	45.0	55.0
Females	32.5	42.5

* Weight load in pounds

PROGRAM 6.4

Recommended program of strength exercise for the fourth week of training.

Exercise order	Training sets	Training repetitions	Training speed[‡]
1. Leg press	1	8-12	2/4
2. Hip adductor	1	8-12	2/4
3. Hip abductor	1	8-12	2/4
4. Decline press	1	8-12	2/4
5. Compound row	1	8-12	2/4
6. Overhead press*	1	8-12	2/4
7. Low back	1	8-12	2/4
8. Abdominal	1	8-12	2/4

*New exercise this week
[‡]Up and down in seconds

Month One, Week Four

During the fourth week of training, you can add another upper body exercise. The recommended addition is the overhead press machine, a linear exercise that uses the deltoids and triceps. Program 6.4 lists the recommended exercise order, and table 6.7 shows the major muscle groups addressed by these eight exercises. As you can see, you are now working on all but one of the major muscle groups.

Do one set of 8 to 12 repetitions with each exercise. When you can reach 12 repetitions, increase your training resistance by about 5 percent. Typical starting weight loads for the overhead press exercise based on your age and gender are listed in table 6.8.

MONTH TWO

During the second month of training you may add two more exercises for the upper body, both performed on the weight-assisted chin-dip machine.

Table 6.7 Muscles addressed by eight Nautilus machines: Month one, week four.	
Major muscle group	**Machine**
1. Quadriceps	Leg press
2. Hamstrings	Leg press
3. Hip adductors	Hip adductor
4. Hip abductors	Hip abductor
5. Pectoralis major	Decline press
6. Latissimus dorsi	Compound row
7. Deltoids	Overhead press
8. Biceps	Compound row
9. Triceps	Decline press
	Overhead press
10. Low back	Low back
11. Abdominals	Abdominal
12. Neck	X X X

Table 6.8 Typical beginning weight loads for selected Nautilus machine by age and gender.	
Age group	**Overhead press (pounds)**
20-29	
Males	65.0
Females	35.0
30-39	
Males	60.0
Females	35.0
40-49	
Males	55.0
Females	32.5
50-59	
Males	50.0
Females	32.5
60-69	
Males	45.0
Females	30.0
70-79	
Males	40.0
Females	30.0

The weight-assisted chin-dip machine gives you two excellent exercises that use four major muscle areas of the upper body. The chin-up is a linear exercise that stresses the latissimus dorsi and biceps. These muscles are responsible for nearly all pulling movements. The bar-dip is a linear exercise that uses the pectoralis major and triceps. These muscles produce force for most pushing movements as well as striking actions such as a tennis stroke, golf drive, and volleyball serve. Program 6.5 lists the recommended exercise order. These nine machines use almost all of the major muscle groups (see table 6.9).

You only need to do one set of 8 to 12 repetitions with each exercise. As usual, when you can complete 12 repetitions, increase your training resistance by about 5 percent. Table 6.10 shows typical starting weight loads for these new exercises based on your age and gender.

MONTH THREE

Expand your program to include three additional machines during the third month of training. These are the 4-way neck machine, the preacher curl machine, and the triceps extension machine. The 4-way neck machine offers four rotary exercises for the neck muscles, the most important of which are neck flexion and neck extension. A strong neck reduces the risk of injury and degenerative problems in this vulnerable area of

PROGRAM 6.5

Recommended program of strength exercise for the second month of training.

Exercise order	Training sets	Training repetitions	Training speed[‡]
1. Leg press	1	8-12	2/4
2. Hip adductor	1	8-12	2/4
3. Hip abductor	1	8-12	2/4
4. Decline press	1	8-12	2/4
5. Compound row	1	8-12	2/4
6. Overhead press	1	8-12	2/4
7. Low back	1	8-12	2/4
8. Abdominal	1	8-12	2/4
9. Chin-dip*	1	8-12	2/4

*New exercise this month
[‡]Up and down in seconds

the body. The preacher curl machine provides rotary exercise for the biceps, while the triceps extension machine provides rotary exercise for the triceps. These machines strengthen the arm muscles in a full range. Program 6.6 lists the recommended exercise order. These 12 machines address all of the major muscle groups with extra attention to the upper body (see table 6.11).

Perform one set of 8 to 12 repetitions with each exercise. When you can complete 12 repetitions, increase your training resistance by about 5 percent. Table 6.12 shows typical starting weight loads for these new exercises based on your age and gender.

MONTH FOUR

Congratulations on completing three months of regular strength workouts! You have made it through the most difficult training phase and you should be noticeably stronger at this point. After 12 weeks of strength training, it is time to change a few of the exercises. To avoid overtraining,

Table 6.9 Muscles addressed by nine Nautilus machines: Month two.	
Major muscle group	**Machine**
1. Quadriceps	Leg press
2. Hamstrings	Leg press
3. Hip adductors	Hip adductor
4. Hip abductors	Hip abductor
5. Pectoralis major	Decline press
	Weight-assisted chin-dip
6. Latissimus dorsi	Compound row
	Weight-assisted chin-dip
7. Deltoids	Overhead press
8. Biceps	Compound row
	Weight-assisted chin-dip
9. Triceps	Decline press
	Overhead press
	Weight-assisted chin-dip
10. Low back	Low back
11. Abdominals	Abdominal
12. Neck	X X X

Table 6.10
Typical beginning weight loads for the Nautilus chin-dip machine by age and gender.

Age group	Chin-up*	Bar-dip*
20-29		
Males	40	40
Females	55	55
30-39		
Males	45	45
Females	60	60
40-49		
Males	50	50
Females	65	65
50-59		
Males	55	55
Females	70	70
60-69		
Males	60	60
Females	75	75
70-79		
Males	65	65
Females	80	80

Percentage of body weight

substitute three new rotary machines for three of the previously used linear machines. Replace the decline press machine with the chest machine, the compound row machine with the super pullover machine, and the shoulder press machine with the lateral raise machine. These changes give more specific training to the torso muscles (pectoralis major, latissimus dorsi, and deltoids), while preventing overtraining of the arm muscles (biceps and triceps). In addition, the new exercises require new muscle response patterns that enhance strength building by activating different muscle fibers. Program 6.7 lists the suggested exercise order. Table 6.13 shows the major muscle groups used by the new group of 12 machines.

Continue to perform one set of 8 to 12 repetitions with each exercise. When you can complete 12 repetitions, increase your training resistance by about 5 percent. Table 6.14 lists typical starting weight loads for these new exercises based on your age and gender.

MONTH FIVE

You are now ready to change the lower body exercises. Substitute the leg extension machine and seated leg curl machine for the leg press machine. Although the leg press is a productive means for working the quadriceps and hamstrings simultaneously, it is time to address these impor-

PROGRAM 6.6

Recommended program of strength exercise for the third month of training.

Exercise order	Training sets	Training repetitions	Training speed‡
1. Leg press	1	8-12	2/4
2. Hip adductor	1	8-12	2/4
3. Hip abductor	1	8-12	2/4
4. Decline press	1	8-12	2/4
5. Compound row	1	8-12	2/4
6. Overhead press	1	8-12	2/4
7. Preacher curl*	1	8-12	2/4
8. Triceps extension*	1	8-12	2/4
9. Low back	1	8-12	2/4
10. Abdominal	1	8-12	2/4
11. 4-way neck*	1	8-12	2/4
12. Chin-dip	1	8-12	2/4

*New exercises this month
‡Up and down in seconds

tant muscles individually. The leg extension is a rotary exercise that targets the quadriceps, and the seated leg curl is a rotary exercise for the hamstrings.

This month you may also replace the abdominal machine with the rotary torso machine. The rotary torso machine uses two separate exercise movements that emphasize the external and internal oblique muscles around your sides. This machine also involves the abdominal muscles, providing comprehensive conditioning for your midsection area. Program 6.8 lists the recommended exercise order. Table 6.15 shows the major muscle groups used.

Perform one set of 8 to 12 repetitions with each exercise. When you

Table 6.11 Muscles addressed by 12 Nautilus machines: Month three.	
Major muscle group	**Machine**
1. Quadriceps	Leg press
2. Hamstrings	Leg press
3. Hip adductors	Hip adductor
4. Hip abductors	Hip abductor
5. Pectoralis major	Decline press
	Weight-assisted chin-dip
6. Latissimus dorsi	Compound row
	Weight-assisted chin-dip
7. Deltoids	Overhead press
8. Biceps	Compound row
	Weight-assisted chin-dip
	Preacher curl
9. Triceps	Decline press
	Weight-assisted chin-dip
	Triceps extension
	Overhead press
10. Low back	Low back
11. Abdominals	Abdominal
12. Neck	4-way neck

Table 6.12
Typical beginning weight loads for selected Nautilus machines by age and gender.

Age group	Neck flexion*	Neck extension*	Preacher curl*	Triceps extension*
20-29				
Males	45.0	50.0	60.0	60.0
Females	30.0	35.0	32.5	32.5
30-39				
Males	42.5	47.5	55.0	55.0
Females	27.5	32.5	30.0	30.0
40-49				
Males	40.0	45.0	50.0	50.0
Females	25.0	30.0	27.5	27.5
50-59				
Males	37.5	42.5	45.0	45.0
Females	22.5	27.5	25.0	25.0
60-69				
Males	35.0	40.0	40.0	40.0
Females	20.0	25.0	22.5	22.5
70-79				
Males	32.5	37.5	35.0	35.0
Females	20.0	25.0	20.0	20.0

Weight load in pounds

can complete 12 repetitions, increase your training resistance by about 5 percent. Table 6.16 shows typical starting weight loads for these new exercises based on your age and gender.

MONTH SIX

You may now replace the weight-assisted chin-dip machine with exercises for muscle groups not yet addressed. This will keep you from overtraining certain muscles and will allow you to add some previously untrained muscles to your exercise program. Although not generally considered major muscle groups, the calf and forearm muscles are important for both everyday function and athletic performance. The seated calf machine uses the gastrocnemius and soleus of the lower leg, while the super forearm machine targets the flexor, extensor, and rotator muscles of the forearms. Both machines provide rotary exercise, with the super-forearm machine offering five separate movements for the fore-

PROGRAM 6.7

Recommended program of strength exercise for the fourth month of training.

Exercise order	Training sets	Training repetitions	Training speed[‡]
1. Leg press	1	8-12	2/4
2. Hip adductor	1	8-12	2/4
3. Hip abductor	1	8-12	2/4
4. Chest*	1	8-12	2/4
5. Super pullover*	1	8-12	2/4
6. Lateral raise*	1	8-12	2/4
7. Preacher curl	1	8-12	2/4
8. Triceps extension	1	8-12	2/4
9. Low back	1	8-12	2/4
10. Abdominal	1	8-12	2/4
11. 4-way neck	1	8-12	2/4
12. Chin-dip	1	8-12	2/4

* New exercises this month
[‡] Up and down in seconds

arm muscles. Do one set of each exercise, starting with a resistance that permits at least 8 repetitions for each exercise and increasing the weight load by about 5 percent when you can complete 12 repetitions.

After half a year of standard strength exercise, you must periodically change some exercises for better training results. New exercises activate different muscle fibers which helps you build more strength. For ex-

Table 6.13
Muscles addressed by 12 Nautilus machines: Month four.

Major muscle group	Machine
1. Quadriceps	Leg press
2. Hamstrings	Leg press
3. Hip adductors	Hip adductor
4. Hip abductors	Hip abductor
5. Pectoralis major	Chest
	Weight-assisted chin-dip
6. Latissimus dorsi	Super pullover
	Weight-assisted chin-dip
7. Deltoids	Lateral raise
8. Biceps	Preacher curl
	Weight-assisted chin-dip
9. Triceps	Triceps extension
	Weight-assisted chin-dip
10. Low back	Low back
11. Abdominals	Abdominal
12. Neck	4-way neck

Table 6.14
Typical beginning weight loads for selected Nautilus machines by age and gender.

Age group	Chest*	Super pullover*	Lateral raise*
20-29			
Males	60.0	65.0	55.0
Females	37.5	40.0	35.0
30-39			
Males	57.5	62.5	52.5
Females	35.0	37.5	32.5
40-49			
Males	55.0	60.0	50.0
Females	32.5	35.0	30.0
50-59			
Males	52.5	57.5	47.5
Females	30.0	32.5	27.5
60-69			
Males	50.0	55.0	45.0
Females	27.5	30.0	25.0
70-79			
Males	47.5	52.5	42.5
Females	25.0	27.5	22.5

*Weight load in pounds

ample, the 10° chest machine, 40° chest machine, and incline press machine each provide an excellent workout for the pectoralis major muscles. The behind-the-neck machine and torso arm machine each provide an excellent workout for the latissimus dorsi muscles. The rowing back machine targets the upper back and deltoids, while the neck and shoulder machine effectively addresses these muscle groups. The lower abdominal machine gives another means for working the midsection and hip flexor muscles. As you can see, many choices of exercises exist for each muscle group. Just be sure to include all of your major muscle groups when redesigning your strength training program. Try to achieve balanced muscular development without overemphasizing or underemphasizing any area of your body. Program 6.9 offers a sample exercise program for the sixth month of strength training.

PROGRAM 6.8

Recommended program of strength exercise for the fifth month of training.

Exercise order	Training sets	Training repetitions	Training speed[‡]
1. Leg extension*	1	8-12	2/4
2. Seated leg curl*	1	8-12	2/4
3. Hip adductor	1	8-12	2/4
4. Hip abductor	1	8-12	2/4
5. Chest	1	8-12	2/4
6. Super pullover	1	8-12	2/4
7. Lateral raise	1	8-12	2/4
8. Preacher curl	1	8-12	2/4
9. Triceps extension	1	8-12	2/4
10. Low back	1	8-12	2/4
11. Rotary torso*	1	8-12	2/4
12. 4-way neck	1	8-12	2/4
13. Chin-dip	1	8-12	2/4

*New exercises this month
[‡]Up and down in seconds

Table 6.15
Muscles addressed by 13 Nautilus machines: Month five.

Major muscle group	Machine
1. Quadriceps	Leg extension
2. Hamstrings	Seated leg curl
3. Hip adductors	Hip adductor
4. Hip abductors	Hip abductor
5. Pectoralis major	Chest
	Weight-assisted chin-dip
6. Latissimus dorsi	Super pullover
	Weight-assisted chin-dip
7. Deltoids	Lateral raise
8. Biceps	Preacher curl
	Weight-assisted chin-dip
9. Triceps	Triceps extension
	Weight-assisted chin-dip
10. Low back	Low back
11. Abdominals	Rotary torso
12. Neck	4-way neck

Table 6.16
Typical beginning weight loads for selected Nautilus machines by age and gender.

Age group	Leg extension*	Seated leg curl*	Rotary torso*
20-29			
Males	70.0	70.0	70.0
Females	42.5	42.5	42.5
30-39			
Males	65.0	65.0	65.0
Females	40.0	40.0	40.0
40-49			
Males	60.0	60.0	60.0
Females	37.5	37.5	37.5
50-59			
Males	55.0	55.0	55.0
Females	35.0	35.0	35.0
60-69			
Males	50.0	50.0	50.0
Females	32.5	32.5	32.5
70-79			
Males	45.0	45.0	45.0
Females	30.0	30.0	30.0

*Weight load in pounds

SUMMARY

Congratulations on half a year of regular strength exercise! The sample six-month strength training program provides a framework for systematically developing higher levels of muscular fitness. It begins with three basic machines that address the most important muscle groups, gradually adding more exercises to include all of your major muscles, then substituting different exercises to ensure progressive strength development without stagnation. This is not the only program that will work with Nautilus machines, but it does give you a sound and sensible exercise progression for safe and productive strength training. Following the recommended training program provides the building blocks to develop a strong musculoskeletal system.

PROGRAM 6.9

Possible program of strength exercise for the sixth month and beyond.

Exercise order	Training sets	Training repetitions	Training speed‡
1. Leg extension	1	8-12	2/4
2. Seated leg curl	1	8-12	2/4
3. Hip adductor	1	8-12	2/4
4. Hip abductor	1	8-12	2/4
5. Seated calf*	1	8-12	2/4
6. 10° chest*	1	8-12	2/4
7. Behind-the-neck*	1	8-12	2/4
8. Rowing back*	1	8-12	2/4
9. Preacher curl	1	8-12	2/4
10. Triceps extension	1	8-12	2/4
11. Low back	1	8-12	2/4
12. Rotary torso	1	8-12	2/4
13. 4-way neck	1	8-12	2/4
14. Super-forearm*	1	8-12	2/4

*New exercises this month
‡Up and down in seconds

CHAPTER 7

Fitness and Cardiovascular Endurance

When you think about endurance training, are you haunted with images of yourself, gaunt and exhausted, dragging over miles of hot and dusty (or maybe cold and snowy!) roads? For many of us who don't care about being super thin or having exceptional athletic stamina, endurance exercise may be synonymous with unpleasant. But in the next few chapters you will see that endurance exercise need not be boring or painful. A variety of aerobic activities and exercise equipment can add "pep" to your program. And even if your workouts are challenging, you will find that the results are well worth the effort. To prevent injury and discouragement, be sure to read both this chapter and the next before beginning your endurance training.

BENEFITS OF ENDURANCE EXERCISE

Properly performed endurance training has many benefits. Unfortunately, many fitness enthusiasts have done too much aerobic exercise and have suffered the consequences of various overuse injuries. When you balance your training program, however, you should experience both better aerobic fitness and enhanced cardiovascular health. The best approach to endurance exercise is performing enough aerobic activity to promote cardiovascular benefits—but not enough to cause musculoskeletal problems. Let's look more closely at the well-documented reasons endurance exercise is so important to a healthy lifestyle.

Physical Capacity

The most obvious outcome of regular endurance exercise is the ability to do more vigorous aerobic activity for longer periods of time. If you are out of shape, you may find it difficult at first to complete even five minutes of light aerobic activity. But as you gradually increase the activity demands, your body adapts and you can exercise at a faster pace for a longer time. Your greater capacity for walking, running, cycling, skating, and stepping makes endurance exercise a worthwhile endeavor.

Cardiovascular Health

Because heart disease accounts for almost half of all deaths in the United States and a substantial percentage of deaths elsewhere, many of us are concerned about our cardiovascular health (1). One of the best ways to avoid cardiovascular illness is to develop and maintain a high level of cardiovascular fitness. Sedentary people have about twice the risk of heart disease as physically active people (2). Actually, being physically inactive increases your risk of heart disease just as much as having high blood pressure, having high blood cholesterol, or smoking cigarettes (3). But even if you have one or more of these risk factors, being in good physical condition can reduce your risk of a heart attack, as shown in figure 7.1 (4). Perhaps more importantly, people in poor physical condi-

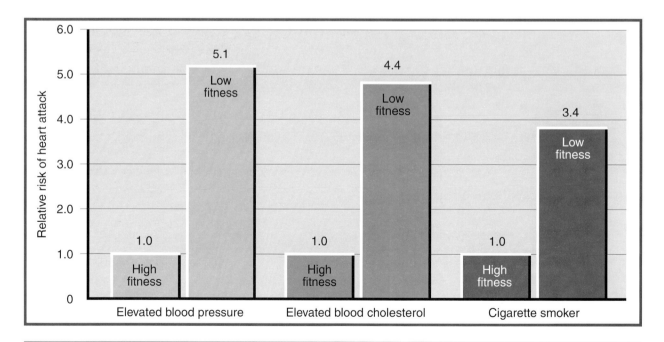

Fig. 7.1 Relative risk of heart attack for 2,779 male public safety officers with cardiovascular risk factors categorized by fitness level.

Reprinted, with permission, from Peters, R.K., L.D. Cady, Jr., D.P. Bischoff et al. 1983. Physical fitness and subsequent myocardial infarction in healthy workers. *JAMA* 249: 3052-3056.

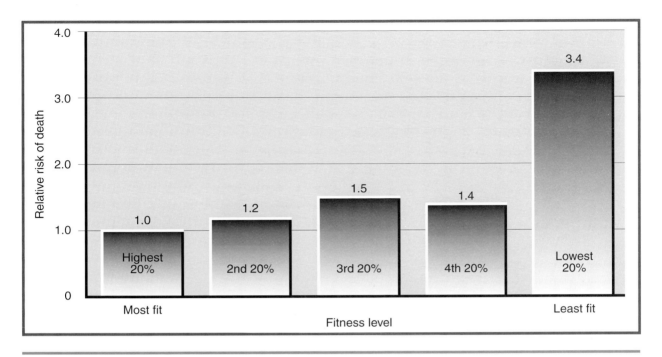

Fig. 7.2 Relative risk of death for 10,244 middle-aged men categorized by fitness level.

Reprinted, with permission, from Blair, S.N., H.W. Kohl, III, D.G. Paffenbarger, Jr. et al. 1989. Physical fitness and all-cause mortality: A prospective study of healthy men and women. *JAMA* 262: 2395-2401.

tion have over three times the risk of death from heart disease and other causes as people with high fitness levels, as illustrated in figure 7.2 (5).

To improve your cardiovascular fitness, you need to do at least 20 minutes of aerobic activity, three nonconsecutive days a week (6). This is a reasonable time commitment in exchange for enjoying a more active lifestyle and better cardiovascular health.

Cardiovascular Function

Many cardiovascular benefits result from regular endurance exercise (7). These positive physiological changes take place in the heart, the circulatory system, and the blood (see table 7.1). Endurance exercise increases your heart's stroke volume and decreases your heart rate, making your heart a stronger pump. A greater stroke volume en-

Table 7.1
Beneficial cardiovascular adaptations associated with regular endurance exercise.*

1. Heart becomes a stronger pump:
   - Stroke volume increases (heart pumps more blood each beat)
   - Heart rate decreases (heart beats less frequently)
   - Cardiac output increases (heart's pumping capacity improves)

2. Circulatory system becomes more efficient in function:
   - Size of blood vessels increases (more blood-carrying capacity)
   - Number of blood vessels increases (better blood distribution)
   - Tone of blood vessels increases (better blood control)

3. Blood becomes a better transporter:
   - Blood volume increases (more transporting capacity)
   - Number of red blood cells increases (more oxygen-carrying capacity)
   - Mass of red blood cells increases (more oxygen-carrying capacity)
   - Platelet stickiness decreases (reduced risk of blood clots)

*Data from Fox, S.M., J.P. Naughton, and P.A. Gorman. 1972. Physical activity and cardiovascular health. *Modern Concepts of Cardiovascular Health* 41: 20.

ables your heart to pump more blood every time it beats. A slower heart rate allows your heart to rest longer and to fill more completely with blood between beats.

After several weeks of regular endurance exercise, you should have a reduced resting heart rate. When you consider that an untrained heart beats about 75 times per minute and that a trained heart beats about 55 times per minute, the savings are almost 30,000 heart beats per day! And that means a lot less wear and tear on your most important muscle.

Your circulatory system responds to endurance exercise by becoming more efficient. The blood vessels increase in size, number, and tone. Larger blood vessels carry more blood to the working muscles, including the heart. More blood vessels distribute blood better within the working muscles, including the heart. Toned blood vessels respond to your body's physical demands better, reducing blood flow to inactive areas and increasing blood flow to the working muscles as needed. These circulatory system changes may reduce resting blood pressure and enhance cardiovascular function.

Endurance exercise also changes your blood for the better. First, regular aerobic activity increases your blood volume, expanding its transporting capacity. Second, it increases the number and size of the red blood cells, enhancing your blood's oxygen-carrying capacity. Third, endurance exercise decreases stickiness among blood platelets, reducing the risk of blood clots.

Although many other cardiovascular improvements result from aerobic activity, Learning about these key benefits should encourage you to do some endurance training. Exercise that makes your heart a stronger pump, your circulatory system more efficient, and your blood a better transporter is certainly worth doing.

Other Health Benefits

Statistics show that we are all at risk when it comes to cardiovascular disease. Therefore, we should make some effort to improve our chances for good health and long life. The most significant coronary risk factors include high blood pressure, high blood cholesterol, cigarette smoking, obesity, glucose intolerance, and psychological stress. Fortunately, regular endurance exercise may help in all of these areas.

Let's start with high blood pressure. Regular endurance exercise effectively reduces both systolic and diastolic blood pressure (see figure 7.3). This is true for endurance exercise alone and in combination with strength training (8-10).

Elevated blood cholesterol levels may also be lowered slightly by regular endurance training. More importantly, endurance exercise has consistently resulted in better ratios of good cholesterol (HDL) to bad cholesterol (LDL), which leads to more desirable lipid profiles (11).

Although aerobic activity does not automatically cause a person to stop smoking, it may influence smoking behavior. At least one study has demonstrated that those who exercise are less likely to smoke than those who don't exercise (12). Smoking and endurance activity are certainly incompatible behaviors, especially if one exercises regularly.

Over one-third of adult Americans are classified as obese (13). In addition to being a cardiovascular risk factor itself, obesity is closely associated with other coronary problems. While dieting can reduce body fat, it also has the undesirable effect of reducing lean tissue. The best fat loss and body composition changes result when you combine dieting with exercise (14-15). As presented in chapter 2, you can achieve a better body composition by doing strength and endurance exercise. After eight weeks of strength and endurance training, adult participants added 3.0 pounds of muscle and lost 8.5 pounds of fat, for an 11.5 pound improvement in body composition (16). Without a doubt, regular endurance exercise can play a significant role in reducing body fat.

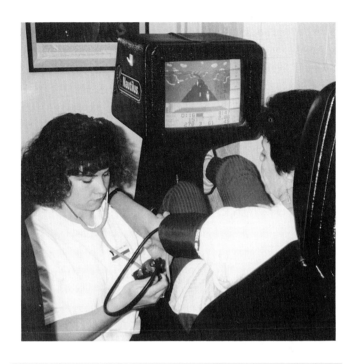

Fig. 7.3 Endurance exercise may help reduce elevated blood pressure.

Glucose intolerance is associated with insulin resistance in our body tissues, which may lead to Type II diabetes and heart disease. Fortunately, Type II diabetes responds favorably to endurance training. Exercise sessions appear to decrease insulin resistance and increase glucose utilization, lessening the risk of glucose intolerance problems (17).

Psychological stress also contributes to cardiovascular risk (18). While research has not proven the positive effects of endurance exercise on psychological stress, most physiologists, psychologists, and fitness enthusiasts agree that physical activity does a good job of reducing the tensions created by daily living.

Other Benefits

You should notice some other benefits from regular aerobic activity. These include improved sleep, digestion, and elimination (7). In addition, people who endurance train often report not only higher levels of energy for performing their exercise sessions but also for doing other physical activities such as gardening, golf, tennis, and skiing (see figure 7.4).

Since your heart functions as the fuel pump for your body, a well-conditioned cardiovascular system enhances the energy supply to your muscles. This helps your muscles to work better and longer, with less effort and faster recovery. When you combine strength and endurance exercise, the improvements in both muscular and cardiovascular fitness make a remarkable difference in your physical capacity. You may wonder how you were able to function adequately before you became fit.

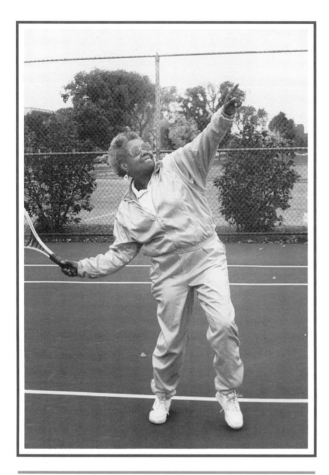

Fig. 7.4 Cardiovascular fitness enables you to do many outdoor activities more easily.

ENDURANCE TRAINING OPTIONS

Now let's look at the many training activities available for designing a workout program. The most popular indoor endurance exercises include treadmill walking and jogging, stationary cycling, stepping machines, and skating machines. Outside the workout room, running, bicycling, swimming, and in-line skating are among the favorites.

In addition to a variety of exercise activities, you can choose from three endurance training methods. The first and most common exercise procedure is steady pace training. The second and the most productive exercise procedure is interval training. The third—and most comprehensive—exercise procedure is cross-training.

Steady Pace Training

Most people prefer steady pace training because it demands a consistent and comfortable exercise effort. For instance, you may find it convenient to walk at a specific speed, such as three and one-half miles an hour. This facilitates a steady heart rate response at a given training level, making it an excellent way to exercise safely. Walking at 3.5 miles an hour may raise your heart rate to the appropriate conditioning level, which will be discussed in chapter 8. As you become more fit, you may need to increase your pace to four miles an hour to have the same training effect.

Steady pace training should not be too easy nor too hard. Make it vigorous enough to improve your cardiovascular system but not so strenuous that it raises your risk of injury. As a rule, if you are able to converse in short sentences during steady pace training, you are probably exercising at a moderate effort level.

Interval Training

Interval training divides your endurance exercise session into harder and easier segments. For example, you may be able to run four miles at a 9.5-minute-a-mile pace, but you would like to improve to a 9-minute-

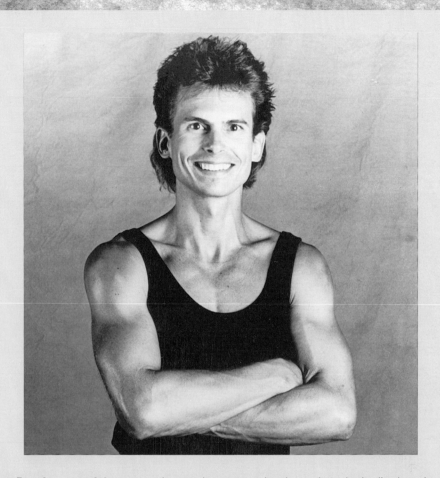

Douglas Brooks, one of the country's premier personal trainers, is truly the "trainers' trainer." He lectures and conducts workshops on exercise physiology, strength training, and personal training throughout the United States and abroad. A personal trainer of the stars, Douglas also appears in training videos of his own and on QVC and the Cable Health Club Network.

Douglas is widely sought after as an expert in strength training, yet he also emphasizes endurance training in his own routine. He tries to challenge all the fitness markers: cardiorespiratory fitness, muscular strength and endurance, and flexibility. Most days of the week, Douglas achieves at least 30 minutes of cardiorespiratory activity. He enjoys outdoor activities, from hiking and swimming to skiing. Using a traditional indoor health club as well, Douglas comments, "Variety is important in my approach to fitness. We need to keep our bodies guessing, the results coming, and our minds fresh. The mental break and infusion of positive energy I get from each effort is the ultimate motivator."

a-mile pace. Try alternating harder and easier mile segments for the four-mile distance. That is, run the first mile in 9 minutes, the second mile in 10 minutes, the third mile in 9 minutes, and the fourth mile in 10 minutes.

Although your total running time is the same, the effort you put into your workout and the benefits you gain will be greater in the interval workout. This is because the 9-minute-mile segments place higher demands on your cardiovascular system, while the 10-minute-mile segments give you recovery intervals, helping you to maintain a desirable overall heart rate response. Interval training provides better cardiovascular conditioning while preparing your body for a faster running pace.

Another physiological advantage of interval training is that it provides more than one cardiovascular stimulus per training session. Each high-effort training interval has a positive impact on your heart's stroke volume, and helps develop a greater pumping capacity.

A psychological advantage of interval training is the faster than normal training pace. Although the high-effort segments may be relatively brief, they demonstrate greater performance potential, making the usual training pace seem a little less demanding by comparison.

The concept of interval training is fairly simple, yet the training options allow considerable personalization. You have several interval training variations as you progress to higher levels of cardiovascular fitness.

- First, you can increase the exercise effort required during the harder intervals.

- Second, you can increase the exercise effort required during the easier intervals.

- Third, you can increase the length of the harder intervals.

- Fourth, you can decrease the length of the easier intervals.

- Fifth, you can increase the number of hard and easy intervals that you complete during a training session.

Cross-Training

Cross-training is another approach to endurance exercise. While interval training alternates harder and easier segments of the same exercise, cross-training involves more than one exercise activity. For example, a 30-minute cross-training session may include 10 minutes of recumbent cycling, 10 minutes of stepping, and 10 minutes of skating. You may do cross-training exercises at a moderate pace or use higher- and lower-effort intervals throughout the workout. Many endurance athletes cross-train during the off-season to maintain their cardiovascular fitness and avoid overuse injuries (see figure 7.5).

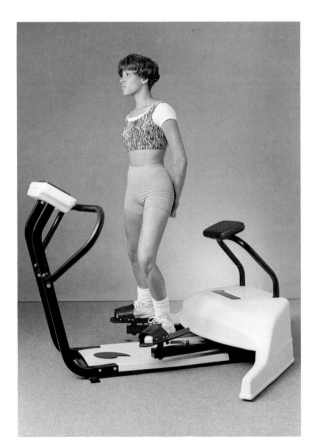

Fig. 7.5 Athletes who compete in summer sports may cross-train by doing running, stepping, cycling, or skating during the winter months.

The advantages of cross-training are two-fold. Psychologically, by frequently changing the exercises, you are less likely to experience boredom during your training sessions. Physiologically, your cardiovascular system receives a training stimulus throughout the entire exercise session as long as you perform each activity with moderate effort. And by using different muscle groups in different activities, you both increase the general conditioning effect and decrease the risk of overuse injuries. For example, recumbent cycling emphasizes the hamstrings, stepping addresses the quadriceps, and skating targets the hip abductors and adductors.

If you prefer to spend an entire exercise session on a single activity, you can apply cross-training on a week-by-week basis. For example, on Monday you may do 30 minutes of recumbent cycling, on Wednesdays—30 minutes of stepping, and on Fridays—30 minutes of skating. Once again, by including three types of endurance exercise you alternate the use of different muscle groups, reducing the risk of overuse injuries. The benefits to your cardiovascular system are similar for each aerobic activity, as long as you follow the basic principles of endurance exercise explained in the next chapter.

SUMMARY

While you should not overdo endurance exercise, appropriate amounts of aerobic activity give you many physiological benefits. Regular endurance exercise improves cardiovascular function, physical capacity, and cardiovascular health. Remember, because the heart serves as the fuel pump for the body, a well-conditioned cardiovascular system enables your muscles to work better and longer, with less effort and faster recovery.

There are three basic exercise procedures for aerobic activity. Steady pace training is characterized by a consistent and comfortable exercise effort. Interval training divides your endurance workout into harder and easier segments to make the exercise sessions more productive. Cross-training combines different aerobic activities within a given workout. By alternating the use of different muscle groups, these briefer exercise segments provide variety, more comprehensive conditioning, and a lower risk of injury. All of the endurance training procedures are effective for cardiovascular conditioning. It is vital, however, that you follow the basic principles of endurance exercise described in the next chapter.

CHAPTER 8

Training
Your Heart

Although endurance exercise can provide many physical benefits, you should not assume that you can do just any aerobic activity program and achieve the level of cardiovascular fitness you want. Because the effectiveness of endurance exercise methods varies considerably, we recommend the same training principles researched by the American College of Sports Medicine (ACSM). These highly respected exercise guidelines provide a solid framework for improving your endurance fitness safely and productively. For maximum cardiovascular benefit, we suggest that you do a variety of aerobic activities that

- use large muscle groups,
- can be maintained continuously, and
- are rhythmic in nature.

EXERCISE SELECTION AND ORDER

Many aerobic activities meet the criteria of continuous large muscle exercise (1). They include walking, jogging, running, cycling, cross-country skiing, aerobic dancing, rope skipping, rowing, stepping, swimming, in-line skating, and endurance sports, such as soccer and basketball.

Most people do one endurance activity at a time, such as a 5-mile run or a 15-mile bicycle ride. But because of the high rate of overuse injuries, single-exercise endurance training is not recommended. Cross-training with two or more aerobic activities is a better alternative because it provides more comprehensive conditioning, has a lower risk of overuse injuries, and is more interesting. Common cross-training exercises include cycling, running, stepping, and skating, as well as other combinations of endurance activities that complement each other.

Don't worry about a specific order for performing cross-training activities. Except for triathletes who must swim first, cycle second, and run third, the exercise order is a matter of personal preference. Each aerobic activity produces about the same benefits for your cardiovascular system but uses different muscle groups. For example, swimming emphasizes the upper body, cycling works on the quadriceps and hamstrings, and skating targets the inner and outer thigh muscles.

Although outdoor activities such as walking and bicycling are attractive options, these may not be the best choices for everyone. Safe outdoor walking or cycling requires sidewalks, bike paths, or roads with little traffic to avoid accidents. Weather and surface conditions, such as rain, snow, or ice, can interfere with your outdoor exercise program. For a variety of control factors, beginners who are overweight or otherwise out of shape usually find well-designed endurance equipment more appropriate. Such equipment provides structural stability and training consistency, with precise exercise conditions that you can repeat or change progressively each workout.

If you are unfit, recumbent cycling is the best activity to initiate your endurance training program (see figure 8.1). First, the recumbent cycle supports your back and body weight, eliminating weightbearing forces that could overstress weak muscles and joints. Second, the recumbent cycle places your body in a more horizontal position, improving blood circulation and cardiovascular function. Third, the recumbent cycle provides electronic resistance that you can adjust to any fitness level, rather than body weight resistance, which may be too much for your present aerobic capacity.

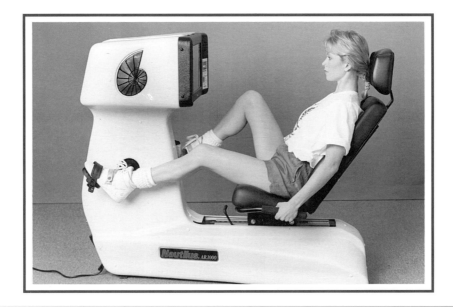

Fig. 8.1 The recumbent cycle provides both body support and great endurance exercise.

The next recommended activity is treadmill walking (see figure 8.2). This is the most natural and least stressful weightbearing exercise. Because walking is mostly a horizontal movement, it is not too demanding on your muscular or cardiovascular system. Of course, you may raise the treadmill incline, walk faster, or progress to jogging as your aerobic condition improves.

Skating provides an excellent follow-up aerobic activity to walking. Like walking, skating primarily involves a horizontal movement pattern that is easy on your joints. Unlike walking, skating emphasizes the inner thigh (adductor) and outer thigh (abductor) muscles. Skating, however, involves virtually all of the leg and hip muscles (see figure 8.3) and is just as effective as cycling and walking for cardiovascular conditioning (2).

Stepping (see figure 8.4) is more demanding than cycling, walking, and skating because its vertical movement pattern lifts your body directly against the force of gravity every step you take (2). You should develop at least a moderate level of cardiovascular conditioning before you add stepping to your exercise program.

Of course, you may do the activity you choose at various effort levels. For example, you may do a low-effort walk on a flat treadmill or a high-effort run on an inclined treadmill. Naturally, you can train longer at a slower pace than you can at a faster pace. Just remember the key to

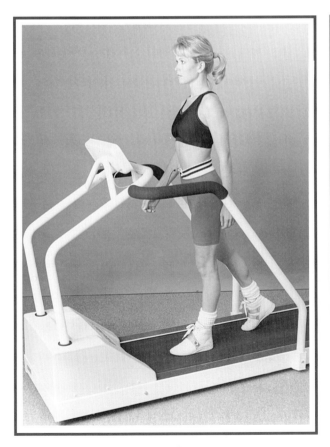

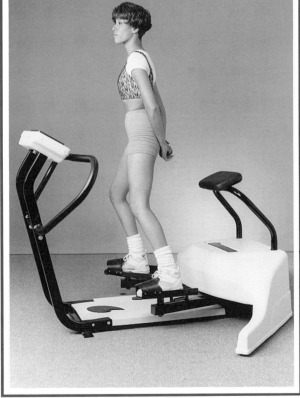

Fig. 8.2 Treadmills offer a constant training pace and controlled conditions for walking and running.

Fig. 8.3 The new skate machine uses the inner and outer thigh muscles.

achieving cardiovascular fitness is following the basic endurance training principles, always using the large muscle groups in continuous and rhythmic movement patterns.

Exercise Frequency

Although endurance exercise affects your muscular system, its primary purpose is cardiovascular conditioning. You should do at least two aerobic workouts a week to improve your cardiovascular fitness (1). Three sessions a week produce almost the same results as five workouts—so more is not necessarily better. Encouraging news for busy people! In fact, training more than three to five days a week increases the risk of injury without adding cardiovascular benefits (3).

For most people, three days of endurance training a week are adequate. If you choose to train more frequently, however, try to limit really challenging workouts to three sessions a week.

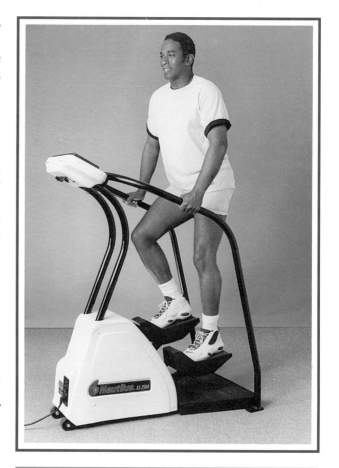

Fig. 8.4 The step machine offers a challenging endurance exercise.

Exercise Duration

Short bursts of exercise can develop muscular strength, but longer workouts of continuous activity are necessary to improve cardiovascular endurance. For example, each set of strength exercise requires about one minute, while a session of endurance activity may take 20 to 60 minutes.

Strength training is high-intensity, low-duration exercise, while endurance training is low-intensity, high-duration exercise. But within certain limits, endurance exercise may vary considerably in intensity and duration. For example, 30 minutes of running and 60 minutes of walking are different aerobic activities that require approximately the same amount of energy (4). When the total work you do is about equal, shorter sessions of faster-paced endurance exercise and longer sessions of slower-paced endurance exercise will give you similar improvements in cardiovascular fitness.

Generally speaking, you should begin with slower-paced aerobic activities that are well within your fitness ability, placing less stress on your body. Start with just a few minutes of endurance exercise and gradually increase the activity duration.

At some point in your training progression, the exercise pace may seem too easy and the exercise duration may seem too long. When this happens, gradually increase your exercise pace and decrease your exercise duration until your training session is more satisfying. Soon you'll be covering the same "ground" in much less time.

While your workout duration is largely a matter of personal preference, it is important to stay within the range of 20 to 60 minutes (1). Doing less than 20 minutes of aerobic activity may decrease the benefits of your training, while completing more than 60 minutes of endurance exercise may increase your risk of overuse injury.

People who perform 20 to 30 minutes of aerobic activity are more likely to stay with their training program than those who attempt 50 to 60 minutes. In our time-pressured society, long training sessions seem more difficult to maintain on a regular basis. Many people find that 20 to 30 minutes of strength training combined with 20 to 30 minutes of endurance training creates a practical and productive program for improving their overall physical fitness.

Exercise Intensity

Exercise intensity is the effort level at which you perform aerobic activity. A simple means for rating your exercise intensity is referred to as the "talk test." If you can talk normally, your effort is most likely low. If you are able to speak only in short sentences, your effort is most likely moderate. But if you are not capable of carrying on a conversation at all, your level of effort is definitely high.

While the talk test provides a reasonable estimate of your training intensity, it is clearly subjective in nature. For example, some people may rate a moderate effort as light, while others may consider a moderate effort to be heavy. For this reason you should use a more objective method of determining your level of effort, at least until you become familiar with these rating relationships.

Because your heart rate is closely related to your training effort, heart rate monitoring is a more precise means of assessing your exercise intensity. Generally speaking, your maximum heart rate may be estimated by subtracting your age from 220. For example, if you are 40 years old, your predicted maximum heart rate is about 180 beats per minute. If you are 50 years old, your predicted maximum heart rate is about 170 beats per minute. As you can see, your maximum heart rate decreases about one beat a year throughout adult life. This is a normal part of the aging process and does not limit your ability to achieve a high level of aerobic fitness. Table 8.1 lists predicted maximum heart rates for men and women between 20 and 90 years of age.

Your maximum heart rate corresponds to an all-out exercise effort in which you are pumping as much oxygen-rich blood as possible to your working muscles. Of course, you can only train at your maximum physical capacity for a short period of time, and such intense exercise is not appropriate for cardiovascular conditioning.

The minimum training intensity for improving your aerobic capacity is approximately 60 percent of your maximum heart rate (1). As your fitness level increases, however, you should train at a higher intensity. If you are in moderate physical condition, you should train at about 70 percent of your maximum heart rate. If you are really fit, exercise at about 80 percent of your maximum heart rate. Check table 8.1 to determine your appropriate exercise heart rate. Of course, you will have to monitor your heart rate periodically during your training session.

Because it is difficult to feel your pulse when you are exercising, simply pause for 10 seconds every 10 minutes during your workout. Place your fingers on your wrist and keep your eyes on your watch as you count every heartbeat for 10 seconds. Multiply by six to determine your training heart rate in beats per minute. For example, if you count 20 beats in 10 seconds, your exercise heart rate is about 120 beats a minute. If you take your pulse for more than 10 seconds, your heart rate may slow down so much that you will underestimate your actual training heart rate.

As you gain experience monitoring your exercise heart rate, you will correlate your heart rate response with your talking ability. That is, you may closely estimate your exercise heart rate based on your subjective assessment of the training effort. Nonetheless, you should periodically check your pulse during exercise (see figure 8.5), because factors other

Table 8.1
Predicted maximum age-related heart rates and selected percentages for training purposes.

	Predicted maximum heart rate (beats per minute)			
Age (years)	60 percent	70 percent	80 percent	100 percent
20	120	140	160	200
25	117	136	156	195
30	114	133	152	190
35	111	129	148	185
40	108	126	144	180
45	105	122	140	175
50	102	119	136	170
55	99	115	132	165
60	96	112	128	160
65	93	108	124	155
70	90	105	120	150
75	87	101	116	145
80	84	98	112	140
85	81	94	108	135
90	78	91	104	130

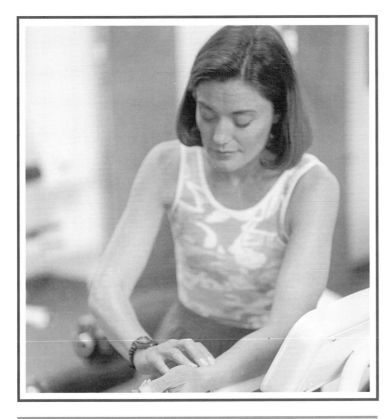

Fig. 8.5 To estimate your exercise heart rate, count your pulse for 10 seconds and multiply by 6.

than activity level may affect your heart rate. For example, high heat or humidity, psychological stress, and physical illness may make your heart work harder than usual at a given exercise pace.

As you become more fit, you may increase your exercise intensity and train at higher effort levels. Just be sure to avoid overtraining and risking overuse injuries. Unless you are a competitive endurance athlete, you need not exercise harder than 80 percent of your maximum heart rate, because you do not gain additional cardiovascular fitness benefits by training at higher heart rate levels (see figure 8.6). After you surpass the beginning exercise level, you should train between 70 to 80 percent of your maximum heart rate for most practical purposes.

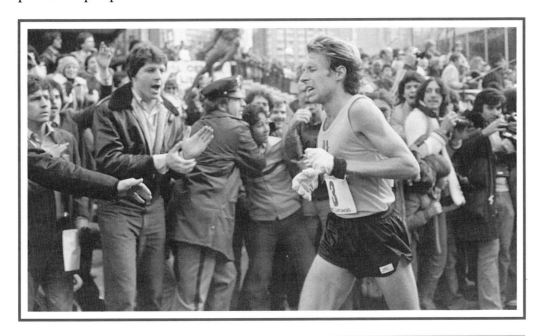

Fig. 8.6 Although you don't need to exercise as hard as Bill Rodgers (above) for fitness, you may enjoy outdoor running in good weather as your cardiovascular endurance improves.

SUMMARY

Remember the general principles of endurance exercise when you select workout activities and determine your training frequency, duration, and intensity. To best condition your cardiovascular system, be sure to choose aerobic activities that use large muscle groups, can be maintained continuously, and are rhythmic in nature. Cycling, walking, jogging, skating, and stepping are all appropriate activities. Just be sure to introduce them in order of their physical demands.

You may endurance train three to five days a week for 20-60 minutes each session. Doing three aerobic workouts a week for 20-30 minutes each session is a safe and practical approach.

Generally, your endurance exercise should require a moderate level of physical effort. You may rate this subjectively by the talk test and objectively through heart rate monitoring. People in poor aerobic condition should train at around 60 percent of their maximum heart rate, while people in moderate aerobic condition should train at around 70 percent of their maximum heart rate, and people in excellent aerobic condition may train at around 80 percent of their maximum heart rate.

CHAPTER 9

Endurance Training Equipment

Have you ever shopped for exercise equipment and been completely confused by all of the models and features that are available? In the area of exercise cycles alone, you may choose an upright or a recumbent model. Some cycles involve leg movements only, while others include arm movements as well. The pedaling resistance may be provided by rubber brakes, weighted belts, air paddles, or electrical currents. Your cycling difficulty may be changed manually or selected from several preprogrammed courses. And the motivational features may range from a simple speedometer to a virtual reality cycling landscape. No wonder choosing the right equipment for your endurance exercise program is so difficult. Use aerobic exercise equipment that is well-designed, scientifically sound, permits gradual warming up and cooling down, provides a variety of training levels and programs, displays performance feedback, offers user-friendly operation, and has a minimum injury risk.

FOUR TYPES OF ENDURANCE TRAINING MACHINES

The fitness industry offers many types of endurance exercise equipment, and within each category, there are many variations in design, function, and performance.

163

In this chapter, four popular types of endurance training machines (recumbent cycles, treadmills, skate machines, and steppers) will be discussed.

Recumbent Cycles

The most obvious difference between the more traditional upright cycle and the more recent recumbent cycle is body position. Upright cycles require a vertical posture in contrast to recumbent cycles, which require a more horizontal exercise position. One advantage of the recumbent cycle is back support. Another benefit of the horizontal position is enhanced blood flow from the legs back to the heart. At the same effort level, your heart rate stays slightly lower during recumbent cycling than upright cycling (1). And recumbent cycling stresses both the quadriceps and the hamstrings, while upright cycling emphasizes the quadriceps. This is because recumbent cycling places fairly equal emphasis on knee extension and hip extension.

Well-designed recumbent cycles offer a wide range of exercise levels to accommodate various fitness abilities. They also give you several exercise programs to choose from, ranging from steady pace training to interval training. Of course, don't forget that each exercise program should begin with a progressive warm-up and finish with a gradual cool-down.

Proper positioning on a recumbent cycle is similar to that on an upright cycle. Adjust the seat so that your knee is slightly bent in the extended pedal position (see figure 9.1). Generally speaking, use a pedaling frequency of approximately 80 revolutions per minute.

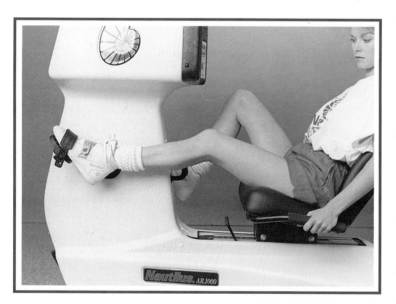

Fig. 9.1 Your knee should be slightly bent when the pedal is in the far position.

Treadmills

There are two basic types of treadmills—those that are self-propelled and those that are motor-driven. Although considerably more expensive, motor-driven treadmills are clearly superior in design, function, and durability. Good motor-driven treadmills have enough horsepower to maintain the desired speed and to keep the track from slipping. The track should be strong and stable to maximize your exercise performance, yet cushioned and resilient to minimize stress on your feet, legs, and lower back. Sturdy handrails and convenient switches are a must for training safety.

The two major program variables in treadmill training are speed and inclination. Well-designed treadmills provide walking and running speeds between 2 and 10 miles an hour. This accommodates the individual who walks at a 30-minute-mile pace, as well as the person who runs at a 6-minute-mile pace.

The greater the treadmill inclination, the greater the exercise effort at a given training speed. For example, if you prefer not to run, you can make your walking workout more challenging by increasing the treadmill inclination. For most practical purposes, treadmills should incline up to seven degrees.

Treadmill walking and running should begin and end with slower-paced warm-up and cool-down segments. The actual conditioning session may consist of steady pace activity or interval exercise, depending on how you change the treadmill speed and inclination.

Keep close to the front panel for proper treadmill positioning. In addition to being in touch with the controls, staying forward reduces your risk of drifting off the back of the track. It is equally important to remain centered on the treadmill track and to turn the motor off before dismounting.

Your exercise posture greatly influences your treadmill performance. Try to walk or run "tall," with normal stride length and natural arm action (see figure 9.2). Avoid short, choppy steps and allow your arms to move smoothly in coordination with your legs. That is, your right arm should move forward and backward with your left leg, and your left arm should move forward and backward with your right leg. Until you become accustomed to walking or running on a moving track, you may need to hold onto the handrail. But as you gain confidence and control, allow your arms to swing freely at your sides to counterbalance your leg movements.

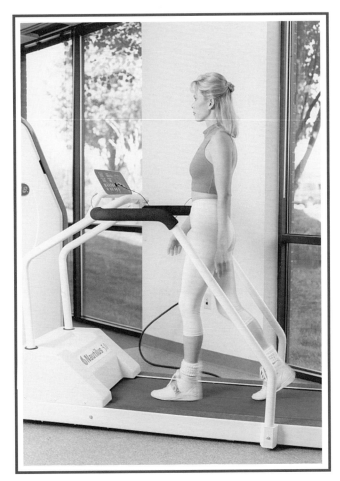

Fig. 9.2 Walk tall with normal stride length on the treadmill.

To maintain the best walking and running form, focus your eyes forward, rather than downward. Keep your shoulders and hips square, without allowing your torso to swing side to side or to shift forward or backward.

Skate Machines

The skate machine is a relatively new addition to the family of aerobic fitness equipment. Its key feature is lateral movement, which targets your inner and outer thighs. This is distinctly different from cycling, walking, running, and stepping, all of which involve up and down movements and use the front and back of your thighs. The skate machine addresses the hip abductor and hip adductor muscles, while other endurance exercise equipment stresses the quadriceps and hamstrings. This makes skating a true cross-training activity. It's also fun!

Another advantage of the skate machine is the horizontal leg action that eliminates landing forces that can jar your feet, legs, and back. The smooth push-glide movements reduce shock and stress to your joints.

In addition to its unique action and muscle involvement, the skate machine provides an effective means of aerobic conditioning. Skating produces nearly the same heart rate and blood pressure readings as cycling and treadmill walking and jogging at a similar effort level (2). In other words, skating offers the same endurance benefits as cycling and treadmill exercising (see table 9.1). And since it uses different muscle groups, it is a good cross-training choice.

As with other forms of aerobic activity, you should begin and end with a few minutes of warm-up and cool-down performed at an easier pace. You may select the actual workout from a variety of exercise programs, or you may design an individualized training program on the control panel.

Although skating form varies among individuals, there are some general guidelines for learning and performing the skate machine. Begin by putting your feet in the skates, placing your hands behind your back, and shifting your weight from side to side. As you master the side-to-side weight shifts, begin to alternately push out and glide back with each

Table 9.1 Heart rate and blood pressure responses at similar effort levels on the cycle, stepper, treadmill, and skate machine (26 subjects).*								
Exercise time (minutes)	Cycle HR	BP	Stepper HR	BP	Treadmill HR	BP	Skate machine HR	BP
4	96	133/76	110	137/74	92	129/74	103	131/71
8	130	153/74	140	148/74	123	143/71	116	145/75
12	138	161/77	143	155/76	126	149/74	127	154/75
16	140	159/76	150	156/72	135	154/73	128	151/76
20	109	135/75	124	135/74	99	134/73	109	135/74
Mean	123	148/76	133	146/74	115	142/73	117	144/74

*Test subjects were 42 years old, having a target heart rate range of 107 to 160 beats per minute.

leg. If you feel unstable at any time, just reach forward and hold the handrail. If you need a rest, simply sit back on the seat.

To maintain the ideal skating form, keep your torso fairly upright and bend your knees as you push off (see figure 9.3). Although your head should remain relatively stable, it's natural for your body to move side-to-side while skating.

Research participants rated the skate machine high in muscular effort and coordination requirements (see table 9.2). In other words, they found both the demands placed on their muscles and the initial learning process challenging. In regard to the cardiovascular effort and overall fitness benefits, the subjects rated skating almost identical to more traditional endurance activities, such as cycling and treadmill work. Used alone, the skate machine is an innovative way to develop aerobic fitness. Used along with other aerobic activities, the skate machine provides a unique form of muscle cross-training and cardiovascular conditioning.

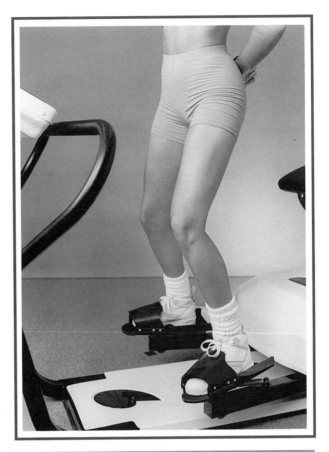

Fig. 9.3 For best results, be sure to bend your knees as you skate.

Steppers

Initially introduced as actual stair-climbing machines with revolving staircases, steppers have become popular endurance training tools. A vigorous exercise, stepping places high demands on your cardiovascular system. It produced higher heart rate responses than cycling, treadmill walking and jogging, and skating when these activities were performed at the same effort

Table 9.2 Subjective rating of selected exercise parameters for similar exercise programs on the cycle, stepper, treadmill, and skate machine (26 subjects).*				
	Cycle	Stepper	Treadmill	Skate machine
Muscular effort	3.3	4.4	2.8	4.1
Cardiovascular effort	3.8	4.6	3.8	3.5
Coordination required	2.2	3.3	2.8	4.6
Overall fitness benefit	3.8	4.4	3.9	3.7
Exercise satisfaction	3.8	4.2	3.6	3.7
*1 = low, 5 = high				

level (table 9.1). This is because stepping requires lifting your body weight vertically, which uses more energy than most other endurance exercises. Research participants rated stepping higher than other aerobic activities for both muscular and cardiovascular effort, which may make it more appropriate for intermediate exercisers than for beginners (see table 9.2). You may select a steady pace step program or a more challenging interval training program.

Step machines fall into two general categories based on their movement mechanics. Independent steppers have separated foot pedals that work independently of each other, with neither foot pedal influencing the action of the other. Dependent steppers have connected foot pedals, that work in coordination. In other words, as the left foot pedal moves upward, the right foot pedal moves downward and vice versa. But since the foot pedal arrangement has little affect on the cardiovascular benefits or energy requirements of stepping, the choice between independent or dependent step machines is largely a matter of personal preference.

Perhaps more important is the step movement pattern. Because you may take thousands of steps during an exercise session, the movement forces should be directed through your lower leg, rather than at various angles to your shin bone (tibia). Step machines that incorporate a four-bar linkage system are most effective in providing the desired performance pattern and reducing injury risk.

Muscle involvement in stepping is closely related to your exercise technique. The quadriceps and hamstrings provide most of the movement force. But the calf muscles of the lower leg are also involved, particularly if you perform much of the stepping action on your toes.

You may involve the muscles of your upper body if you do not use appropriate stepping posture. Proper stepping form requires a fairly upright posture, using your hands for balance, rather than for body support (see figure 9.4). Avoid leaning forward and unnecessarily stressing your wrists and low back, which is not the intent of stepping exercise. As with walking and running, strive to keep your head up and back straight while stepping.

The depth of your steps should be moderate and comfortable. Just as there is no set stride length for walking and running, there is no set step depth for stepping. Shal-

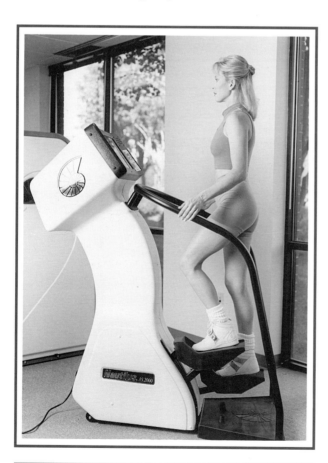

Fig. 9.4 Keep an upright posture and use your hands for balance rather than body support.

low, fast stepping may decrease your muscular work, while deep, slow stepping may increase your risk of injury. A moderate stepping action gives you a reasonable range of movement, effectively involving your muscles, while still maintaining level hips and shoulders.

Because stepping is a demanding physical activity, it is essential to spend the first few minutes warming up and the last few minutes cooling down during each session. Your actual workout may consist of a steady stepping cadence, or a series of high-effort and low-effort intervals. Just be sure to maintain proper form and to remain within your target heart rate zone at all times.

EQUIPMENT SELECTION

The most important consideration in choosing endurance exercise equipment is your personal preference. If you are a lively individual, then you may enjoy the unencumbered feeling of running on a treadmill. If you are overweight or otherwise out of shape, the supportive structure of a recumbent cycle may make more sense as your basic training mode.

Of course, equipment availability may play a major role in your choice of aerobic activity. If you're lucky enough to have access to cycles, treadmills, skate machines, and steppers, then a cross-training program may make your workouts more enjoyable. By performing a combination of endurance exercises each workout, or by changing aerobic activities every training session, you may increase both your motivation and your conditioning.

Choose the modes of endurance exercise that you like best. If you prefer a lower intensity training experience, recumbent cycling may be best for the majority of your endurance workouts. If you like more rhythmic forms of aerobic activity, the skate machine may be the perfect piece of exercise equipment. If you want a high-intensity workout that provides the most training benefit in the least amount of time, and you are already in moderately good shape, try stepping. And if you prefer an activity that combines both rhythm and intensity, treadmill walking and running are good choices.

While all of these aerobic activities involve the larger muscles of the legs, there are some differences in muscle action. Treadmill walking emphasizes the hamstrings in the back of the thigh, stepping targets the quadriceps in the front of the thigh, recumbent cycling works both the hamstrings and quadriceps, and skating addresses the adductors and abductors of the inner and outer thighs.

SUMMARY

You have many choices of endurance exercise. The most popular types of equipment for indoor aerobic training include recumbent cycles, treadmills, skate machines, and steppers. Each of these endurance activities effectively conditions your cardiovascular system, so your choice of exercise equipment is largely a matter of personal preference.

Well-designed aerobic exercise equipment is scientifically sound, permits gradual warming up and cooling down, provides a variety of training levels and programs, displays performance feedback, offers user-friendly operation, and keeps the risk of injury to a minimum. Always use an exercise machine as directed in the manufacturer's handbook and always remember the endurance training principles.

CHAPTER 10

Endurance Training Exercises

Proper performance of endurance exercise involves more than just getting on a piece of aerobic equipment and working out as hard as you can for as long as you can. As with strength training, you should understand certain techniques and be familiar with each machine's features before beginning your exercise program.

GENERAL GUIDELINES

No single method of using the recumbent cycle, treadmill, skate machine, and step machine exists. But it's important to follow general guidelines to ensure safe and productive training.

Regardless of the activity you choose, be sure to check with your personal physician before you exercise. You may also want to consult with a professional exercise instructor if you train at a fitness facility or with a certified personal trainer if you workout at home.

If you dress appropriately for exercise, you will enhance your activity performance and reduce your risk of injury. Proper footwear is first and foremost, especially for weightbearing activities such as walking, jogging, skating, and stepping. You should use supportive, well-cushioned athletic shoes that fit loosely around your toes and snugly around your heels.

Because exercise produces heat, your clothing should allow heat transfer from your body to the environment. Ordinarily, you should wear light, athletic clothing, such as a T-shirt and shorts (see figure 10.1). But if you tend to feel cool in the first few minutes of exercise, wear an athletic suit or sweatshirt that you can easily remove as you warm up and begin to perspire. Just be careful not to overdress, because this prevents perspiration from evaporating. And when you are exercising vigorously, evaporation of perspiration from the skin is essential for releasing your body heat.

Along this same line, it's important to stay well-hydrated throughout your exercise session. Drink plenty of fluids—preferably water—before each workout. To replace water while exercising, drink often from a water bottle at your activity station. Because you probably will lose more water than you can consume during exercise, be sure to continue drinking after your workout. You may substitute fruit juices and sport drinks for water, but you should avoid caffeinated or alcoholic beverages because these dehydrate you. As a rule, you should drink at least eight glasses of water each day.

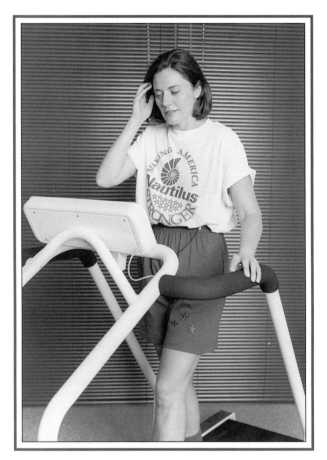

Fig. 10.1 Lightweight athletic clothing facilitates heat transfer from your body to the environment.

Monitoring your training progress is an excellent motivator, so record each exercise session in a training logbook. Keep track of your exercise activity, intensity level, training duration, exercise heart rate, and other pertinent information. Review your logbook whenever you need an extra boost to your morale. When you see how much you have improved, you'll realize how much your training investment has paid off. The logbook also provides valuable information to guide you as you plan progressively more difficult workouts.

TRAINING PROCEDURES

Now you're ready to learn specific training procedures for using endurance exercise equipment. Let's begin with a less stressful form of aerobic activity—recumbent cycling.

Recumbent Cycle

As discussed in chapter 9, the primary difference between the upright and recumbent cycle is that the recumbent bike offers back and neck support. Because your legs are mostly horizontal, it is easier for your cardiovascular system to return blood to your heart. For these reasons, the recumbent cycle is the best choice for overweight or otherwise underconditioned people.

Procedure

1. Adjust the seat so that your knees are slightly bent when your feet are in the extended pedal positions. Slide each foot as far into the pedal strap as is comfortable, with the ball of the foot over the pedal pivot point (see figure 10.2). Make sure your back and hips are fully supported by the seat back. Place your hands across your lap or on the sides of the seat.

2. Turn on the exercise monitor and select an appropriate exercise profile. Choose a program with a progressive warm-up, a gradual cool-down, and a constant training level in between.

3. Adjust the effort level to your current fitness ability. Levels 1, 2, or 3 are recommended for beginners; levels 4, 5, or 6 for intermediate exercisers; and levels 7, 8, or 9 for advanced participants.

4. Adjust the exercise time according to your fitness level. If you're a beginner, stay in the range of 2 to 10 minutes. If you consider yourself moderately fit, exercise for 10 to 20 minutes. If you're in pretty good shape, train for 20 to 30 minutes. Competitive athletes may wish to exercise longer, but if your primary purpose is cardiovascular fitness, you don't need to cycle more than 30 minutes.

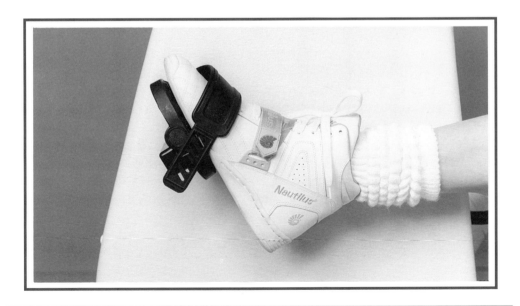

Fig. 10.2 Try to place the ball of your foot directly over the pedal pivot point.

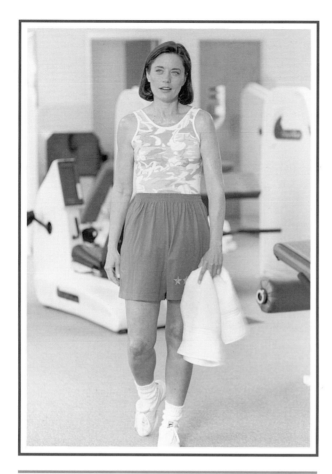

Fig. 10.3 One of the best cool-down activities is walking.

5. Keep your pedaling speed approximately 20 miles an hour or about 80 pedal revolutions a minute. If your bike has a pacer, do your best to stay with the pacer throughout the exercise program.

After completing the course, be sure to cool down with a slower, but still continuous, pedaling action. Push the seat backward to dismount, then walk around to finish your cool-down (see figure 10.3).

Motor-Driven Treadmills

Motor-driven treadmills force you to exercise consistently and keep pace with the moving track. Treadmills without motors make it more difficult for you to maintain a steady walking or jogging pace and may be more stressful on your body. Well-designed motor-driven treadmills do not lose speed, skip, or slip—regardless of your size.

Procedure

Before you begin, note where the handlebars and "Stop" switch are located in case you lose your balance.

1. Straddle the track with your feet on the solid side frames, place one hand on the handlebar, and touch the power switch with your other hand. Push the "Grade Down" button to make sure the treadmill is at zero degrees and completely level. If the treadmill offers preprogrammed exercise programs, select your desired workout.

2. Touch the start switch and the track should begin moving slowly. While holding the handrail, place one foot gently on the track and stride with one leg to feel the movement speed. When comfortable, place both feet on the moving track and walk naturally while still holding the handrail.

3. When you feel confident, let go of the handrail first with one hand and then the other and walk naturally. Be sure to stay in the front portion of the track, close to the handrail and controls. Walk with a moderate stride and an opposing arm action (right leg and left arm move forward together; left leg and right arm move forward together). Try to walk "tall" with your head up and your eyes focused ahead rather than down.

4. At this point you will probably want to walk faster, so touch the speed button to quicken your pace. Be sure to increase the miles per

hour gradually as you progress to your desired training speed. Once you reach four miles an hour, you are walking at a relatively fast 15-minute-mile pace. To further increase your effort, raise the grade slightly so that you are walking uphill. For every treadmill training session, you should warm up and cool down for a few minutes at a slow speed and low grade. For the actual training phase, you should choose a moderate effort level, selecting a track speed and elevation that raises your heart rate to about 70 percent of maximum.

5. If you are in poor condition, try a training duration of 2 to 10 minutes; if you are moderately fit, do 10 to 20 minutes; and if you are very fit, workout for 20 to 30 minutes.

6. As you prepare to finish your exercise session, gradually reduce the speed and grade to the lowest levels, grasp the handrail, and touch the "Stop" switch. Do not dismount the track until it has stopped moving completely.

If at any time you feel uncomfortable, off-balance, or out-of-control, immediately touch the "Stop" switch and the track will gently but quickly stop. As an alternative to a steady pace program, you may perform a variety of interval training workouts. For example, you could do three minutes at a slower than normal pace, followed by three minutes at a faster than normal pace, alternated throughout the exercise session. Whatever training program you use, be sure to advance the controls one unit at a time since the track speed and elevation changes are electronically delayed.

Skate Machine

The skate machine is a true cross-training alternative that shapes up the hip abductor and adductor muscles of the inner and outer thighs. It is a weightbearing activity, yet because of the horizontal leg movements, it doesn't jar your joints. Another unique feature of the skate machine is the side-to-side movement that creates constant air circulation. To succeed on the skate machine, relax, bend your knees, hold your head and torso up, and keep your arms close to your body.

Procedure

1. Place your feet in the skates, stand upright, and select a course that has built-in warm-up and cool-down phases, with a constant training level in between.

2. Select an effort level that matches your present fitness ability. If your fitness level is low, use effort level 1, 2, or 3. If you are moderately fit, use effort level 4, 5, or 6, and if your fitness level is high, train at 7, 8, or 9.

3. Set an appropriate training duration. In general, if you are not very fit, set the time for 2 to 10 minutes; if you are moderately fit, set the time for 10 to 20 minutes; and if you are highly fit, 20 to 30 minutes. If you are a skating enthusiast you may exercise longer, but 30 minutes of continuous endurance exercise provides all of the aerobic benefits you need.

4. Learning to use the skate machine is as simple as swaying gently from side-to-side. Begin by shifting your weight smoothly from your left foot to your right foot and vice versa. Next, bend your knees and push to the outside with alternating legs. The actual movement pattern is to push your right leg to the outside while your left leg remains in the center. As your right leg returns to the center, push your left leg to the outside while your right leg remains in the center. Continue this way and you should soon be skating smoothly.

5. Some people place their hands on their hips, others keep them behind their backs, while still others swing their arms in coordination with their legs. Whichever pattern you choose, you should not hold the handrail while you exercise. But if you lose your balance or feel out-of-control, grasp the handrail to stabilize yourself. As an added safety precaution, you may sit on the padded seat.

6. Like the recumbent cycle, the skate machine stops whenever you do. To get off the machine, simply remove your feet from the skates and walk around to finish your cool-down.

If you prefer a more competitive exercise experience, try to keep pace with the built-in pacer. Your skating cadence, however, is strictly a matter of personal preference.

Stepper

The step machine is similar to climbing stairs without the descending action that can cause muscle soreness. Both dependent and independent steppers require alternating contractions of the large leg muscles. This is a demanding exercise because each step lifts your body weight directly against gravity. The most important technique considerations in stepping are maintaining an upright body position, keeping a light grip on the handrails, and using your entire foot with your knee directly over your foot. Be sure not to lean forward or support your weight with your hands, because this stresses your back and wrists, which may lead to injury.

Procedure

1. Step on the pedals and record your body weight according to the computer prompts.

2. Choose an exercise program that has built-in warm-up and cool-down phases with a constant training pace in between. If your present level of fitness is low, train at effort level 1, 2, or 3; if your present fitness level is moderate, train at effort level 4, 5, or 6; and if your present fitness level is high, try 7, 8, or 9.

3. Select an appropriate exercise duration. Beginners should start with 2 to 10 minutes of exercise; intermediate exercisers may train for 10 to 20 minutes; and advanced exercisers, for 20 to 30 minutes.

4. As you exercise, you may make the workout harder or easier by adjusting the effort and pace controls.

5. Take medium steps and maintain level hips and shoulders. Short steps require less muscle action and decrease the training benefits. Long steps exaggerate your hip movement and increase the risk of injury.

6. After you finish your exercise session, dismount the stepper and walk for a few minutes to finish your cool-down.

SUMMARY

Approach endurance exercise sensibly. A "no gain without pain" attitude may do more harm than good. Before beginning your training program, both consult with your physician and receive exercise instruction from a qualified fitness professional. Dress appropriately to allow heat transfer and drink plenty of water to stay well-hydrated. Keep accurate records of each exercise experience both to motivate yourself and to guide you as you gradually progress to more challenging workouts.

For safe and productive endurance exercise, follow the training recommendations and operational procedures given for each machine. Cross-training gives you variety, while effectively alternating different muscle groups. Interval training efficiently raises your work effort, increasing your conditioning benefits in the same amount of training time.

Be sure to begin each endurance training session with a progressive warm-up, work at a moderate effort level, train for a reasonable duration, stay within your target heart rate zone, and end with a gradual cool-down. Most importantly, train on a regular basis, three to five days a week, unless you are ill or injured.

CHAPTER 11

Six-Month Endurance Training Program

Almost anyone can complete a week or two of aerobic exercise, but it's much more difficult to train regularly and progressively long-term. Many beginners do too much too soon, quickly losing their enthusiasm for training. Rather than becoming regular exercisers, they tend to "yo-yo" between short periods of hard training and long periods of no training. One of the best ways for developing training consistency is to follow a six-month plan of endurance exercise. Just be sure to choose aerobic activities that you enjoy and always exercise within your capabilities.

A SIX-MONTH PROGRAM

There are many training programs that may provide effective endurance exercise and enhance your aerobic fitness. The sample six-month training program gives you a safe, progressive, and productive approach to cardiovascular conditioning, using a three-day-a-week exercise regimen.

Adjust these recommendations to your personal interests and abilities. For example, feel free to repeat a month if you are not ready to progress to the next training level.

Month One

Let's begin with recumbent cycling, the endurance exercise that is easiest to perform and least stressful to your cardiovascular and musculoskeletal systems. Choose an appropriate program with substantial warm-up and cool-down segments, select a low effort level, and begin with a brief exercise duration. Program 11.1 shows a sample training program for your first 12 cycling sessions. It is designed to progressively increase the exercise demands on your body as it gradually becomes better-conditioned.

PROGRAM 11.1

Suggested endurance exercise program during the first month of training, doing recumbent cycling.*

Month One	
Week One	
Monday	Cycle 6-10 minutes at a low effort level, approximately 60 percent of your maximum heart rate.
Wednesday	Cycle 6-10 minutes at a low effort level, approximately 60 percent of your maximum heart rate.
Friday	Cycle 8-12 minutes at a low effort level, approximately 60 percent of your maximum heart rate.
Week Two	
Monday	Cycle 8-12 minutes at a low effort level, approximately 65 percent of your maximum heart rate.

Wednesday	Cycle 10-14 minutes at a low effort level, approximately 65 percent of your maximum heart rate.
Friday	Cycle 10-14 minutes at a low effort level, approximately 65 percent of your maximum heart rate.

Week Three

Monday	Cycle 12-16 minutes at a moderate effort level, approximately 70 percent of your maximum heart rate.
Wednesday	Cycle 12-16 minutes at a moderate effort level, approximately 70 percent of your maximum heart rate.
Friday	Cycle 14-18 minutes at a moderate effort level, approximately 70 percent of your maximum heart rate.

Week Four

Monday	Cycle 14-18 minutes at a moderate effort level, approximately 75 percent of your maximum heart rate.
Wednesday	Cycle 16-20 minutes at a moderate effort level, approximately 75 percent of your maximum heart rate.
Friday	Cycle 16-20 minutes at a moderate effort level, approximately 75 percent of your maximum heart rate.

If this equipment is not available, you may substitute a similar endurance exercise.

Month Two

By the beginning of your second month of training, you should be cycling at a moderate effort level for about 20 minutes a session. This gives you adequate cardiovascular conditioning, and you may continue to progress in this aerobic activity if you like. You may prefer, however, to alternate recumbent cycling with another type of endurance exercise, such as treadmill walking. Because you are now at a higher fitness level, you may begin treadmill walking at a moderate effort level and exercise duration. It is important to warm up and cool down and to use proper form throughout each training session. Your second month of training may include two endurance activities with separate but similar exercise programs (see program 11.2).

PROGRAM 11.2

Suggested endurance exercise program during the second month of training, doing recumbent cycling and treadmill walking.*

Month Two	
Week One	
Monday	Cycle 18-22 minutes at a moderate effort level, approximately 75 percent of your maximum heart rate.
Wednesday	Cycle 18-22 minutes at a moderate effort level, approximately 75 percent of your maximum heart rate.
Friday	Walk 14-18 minutes at a moderate effort level, approximately 75 percent of your maximum heart rate.
Week Two	
Monday	Walk 14-18 minutes at a moderate effort level, approximately 75 percent of your maximum heart rate.

Wednesday	Cycle 20-24 minutes at a moderate effort level, approximately 75 percent of your maximum heart rate.
Friday	Cycle 20-24 minutes at a moderate effort level, approximately 75 percent of your maximum heart rate.

Week Three

Monday	Walk 16-20 minutes at a moderate effort level, approximately 75 percent of your maximum heart rate.
Wednesday	Walk 16-20 minutes at a moderate effort level, approximately 75 percent of your maximum heart rate.
Friday	Cycle 22-26 minutes at a moderate effort level, approximately 75 percent of your maximum heart rate.

Week Four

Monday	Cycle 22-26 minutes at a moderate effort level, approximately 75 percent of your maximum heart rate.
Wednesday	Walk 18-22 minutes at a moderate effort level, approximately 75 percent of your maximum heart rate.
Friday	Walk 18-22 minutes at a moderate effort level, approximately 75 percent of your maximum heart rate.

* *If this equipment is not available, you may substitute similar endurance exercises.*

Month Three

During the third month you may increase both your cycling and walking time to 30 minutes a session. You may also add skating to your exercise program, gradually building up to about 20 minutes of this unique aerobic activity. Remember to warm up and cool down before and after each training session and to work within your target heart rate zone. Program 11.3 gives you a sample exercise program for your third month of aerobic conditioning.

PROGRAM 11.3

Suggested endurance exercise program during the third month of training, doing recumbent cycling, treadmill walking, and skating.*

Month Three	
Week One	
Monday	Cycle 24-28 minutes at a moderate effort level, approximately 75 percent of your maximum heart rate.
Wednesday	Walk 20-24 minutes at a moderate effort level, approximately 75 percent of your maximum heart rate.
Friday	Skate 10-14 minutes at a moderate effort level, approximately 75 percent of your maximum heart rate.
Week Two	
Monday	Cycle 26-30 minutes at a moderate effort level, approximately 75 percent of your maximum heart rate.

| **Wednesday** | Walk 22-26 minutes at a moderate effort level, approximately 75 percent of your maximum heart rate. |
| **Friday** | Skate 12-16 minutes at a moderate effort level, approximately 75 percent of your maximum heart rate. |

Week Three

Monday	Cycle 26-30 minutes at a moderate effort level, approximately 75 percent of your maximum heart rate.
Wednesday	Walk 24-28 minutes at a moderate effort level, approximately 75 percent of your maximum heart rate.
Friday	Skate 14-18 minutes at a moderate effort level, approximately 75 percent of your maximum heart rate.

Week Four

Monday	Cycle 26-30 minutes at a moderate effort level, approximately 75 percent of your maximum heart rate.
Wednesday	Walk 26-30 minutes at a moderate effort level, approximately 75 percent of your maximum heart rate.
Friday	Skate 16-20 minutes at a moderate effort level, approximately 75 percent of your maximum heart rate.

*   If this equipment is not available, you may substitute similar endurance exercises.

Month Four

As you enter your fourth month of endurance training, you should be ready for some stepping exercise. During this month, I recommend alternating less stressful skating workouts and more demanding stepping workouts, with occasional sessions on the recumbent cycle and the treadmill. By the end of the fourth month, you should be comfortable with 30 minutes of cycling, walking, and skating. You should also be capable of completing 24 minutes of stepping at a comfortable effort level. Program 11.4 gives you a sample endurance exercise program for your fourth training month.

PROGRAM 11.4

Suggested endurance exercise program during the fourth month of training, doing recumbent cycling, treadmill walking, skating, and stepping.*

Month Four	
Week One	
Monday	Skate 18-22 minutes at a moderate effort level, approximately 75 percent of your maximum heart rate.
Wednesday	Step 10-14 minutes at a moderate effort level, approximately 75 percent of your maximum heart rate.
Friday	Skate 20-24 minutes at a moderate effort level, approximately 75 percent of your maximum heart rate.
Week Two	
Monday	Step 12-16 minutes at a moderate effort level, approximately 75 percent of your maximum heart rate.

Wednesday	Skate 22-26 minutes at a moderate effort level, approximately 75 percent of your maximum heart rate.
Friday	Step 14-18 minutes at a moderate effort level, approximately 75 percent of your maximum heart rate.

Week Three

Monday	Cycle 26-30 minutes at a moderate effort level, approximately 75 percent of your maximum heart rate.
Wednesday	Step 16-20 minutes at a moderate effort level, approximately 75 percent of your maximum heart rate.
Friday	Skate 24-28 minutes at a moderate effort level, approximately 75 percent of your maximum heart rate.

Week Four

Monday	Step 18-22 minutes at a moderate effort level, approximately 75 percent of your maximum heart rate.
Wednesday	Walk 26-30 minutes at a moderate effort level, approximately 75 percent of your maximum heart rate.
Friday	Step 20-24 minutes at a moderate effort level, approximately 75 percent of your maximum heart rate.

* *If this equipment is not available, you may substitute similar endurance exercises.*

Month Five

After four months of progressive cardiovascular conditioning, you should be ready to periodically add some interval training to your exercise program. This will make your workout more interesting, challenging, and productive than only increasing the duration of each aerobic activity will. As explained in chapter 7, interval training is a way to alternate harder and easier exercise segments within your training program. This keeps your time investment the same but increases your overall exercise intensity, uses more energy, and enhances your training benefits.

During this month, each high-effort and low-effort training interval should be three minutes in length, with five minutes each of warming up and cooling down. Because interval training is more demanding, one interval workout a week is sufficient at this stage of your conditioning program. As shown in program 11.5, the interval training session for each exercise activity is scheduled on Fridays to take advantage of the longer weekend recovery period.

PROGRAM 11.5

Suggested endurance exercise program during the fifth month of training, doing recumbent cycling, treadmill walking, skating, and stepping.*

Month Five	
Week One	
Monday	Step 22-26 minutes at a moderate effort level, approximately 75 percent of your maximum heart rate.
Wednesday	Cycle 26-30 minutes at a moderate effort level, approximately 75 percent of your maximum heart rate.
Friday	Walk 28 minutes using an interval training procedure: 5 minutes warm-up, 60 percent maximum heart rate 3 minutes lower-effort interval, 70 percent maximum heart rate 3 minutes higher-effort interval, 80 percent maximum heart rate 3 minutes lower-effort interval, 70 percent maximum heart rate 3 minutes higher-effort interval, 80 percent maximum heart rate 3 minutes lower-effort interval, 70 percent maximum heart rate 3 minutes higher-effort interval, 80 percent maximum heart rate 5 minutes cool-down, 60 percent maximum heart rate

Week Two

Monday	
	Skate 26-30 minutes at a moderate effort level, approximately 75 percent of your maximum heart rate.
Wednesday	
	Step 24-28 minutes at a moderate effort level, approximately 75 percent of your maximum heart rate.
Friday	
	Cycle 28 minutes using an interval training procedure: 5 minutes warm-up, 60 percent maximum heart rate 3 minutes lower-effort interval, 70 percent maximum heart rate 3 minutes higher-effort interval, 80 percent maximum heart rate 3 minutes lower-effort interval, 70 percent maximum heart rate 3 minutes higher-effort interval, 80 percent maximum heart rate 3 minutes lower-effort interval, 70 percent maximum heart rate 3 minutes higher-effort interval, 80 percent maximum heart rate 5 minutes cool-down, 60 percent maximum heart rate

Week Three

Monday	
	Walk 26-30 minutes at a moderate effort level, approximately 75 percent of your maximum heart rate.
Wednesday	
	Skate 26-30 minutes at a moderate effort level, approximately 75 percent of your maximum heart rate.
Friday	
	Step 28 minutes using an interval training procedure: 5 minutes warm-up, 60 percent maximum heart rate 3 minutes lower-effort interval, 70 percent maximum heart rate 3 minutes higher-effort interval, 80 percent maximum heart rate 3 minutes lower-effort interval, 70 percent maximum heart rate 3 minutes higher-effort interval, 80 percent maximum heart rate 3 minutes lower-effort interval, 70 percent maximum heart rate 3 minutes higher-effort interval, 80 percent maximum heart rate 5 minutes cool-down, 60 percent maximum heart rate

Week Four	
Monday	Cycle 26-30 minutes at a moderate effort level, approximately 75 percent of your maximum heart rate.
Wednesday	Walk 26-30 minutes at a moderate effort level, approximately 75 percent of your maximum heart rate.
Friday	Skate 28 minutes using an interval training procedure: 5 minutes warm-up, 60 percent maximum heart rate 3 minutes lower-effort interval, 70 percent maximum heart rate 3 minutes higher-effort interval, 80 percent maximum heart rate 3 minutes lower-effort interval, 70 percent maximum heart rate 3 minutes higher-effort interval, 80 percent maximum heart rate 3 minutes lower-effort interval, 70 percent maximum heart rate 3 minutes higher-effort interval, 80 percent maximum heart rate 5 minutes cool-down, 60 percent maximum heart rate

* If this equipment is not available, you may substitute similar endurance exercises.

Month Six

Congratulations on completing a progressive aerobic training program up to this point! As you approach one-half year of regular endurance exercise, you may want to expand your cross-training and interval training into a four-day-a-week workout program. Of course, always select the training program that works best for you and feel free to continue your three-day-a-week schedule if this is satisfactory. Program 11.6 shows you how to systematically continue improving in your cardiovascular conditioning program. You should follow this workout schedule as closely as possible during your sixth month of training. If you choose to use different exercises, try to alternate between more stressful and less stressful ones.

PROGRAM 11.6

Suggested endurance exercise program during the sixth month of training, doing recumbent cycling, treadmill walking, skating, and stepping.*

Month Six
Week One

Monday	Walk or jog 26-30 minutes at a moderate effort level, approximately 75 percent of your maximum heart rate.
Wednesday	Cycle 26-30 minutes at a moderate effort level, approximately 75 percent of your maximum heart rate.
Friday	Walk or jog 26-30 minutes at a moderate effort level, approximately 75 percent of your maximum heart rate.
Saturday	Cycle 28 minutes using an interval training procedure: 5 minutes warm-up, 60 percent maximum heart rate 2 minutes lower-effort interval, 70 percent maximum heart rate 4 minutes higher-effort interval, 80 percent maximum heart rate 2 minutes lower-effort interval, 70 percent maximum heart rate 4 minutes higher-effort interval, 80 percent maximum heart rate 2 minutes lower-effort interval, 70 percent maximum heart rate 4 minutes higher-effort interval, 80 percent maximum heart rate 5 minutes cool-down, 60 percent maximum heart rate

Week Two

Monday	Step 26-30 minutes at a moderate effort level, approximately 75 percent of your maximum heart rate.

Wednesday	Skate 26-30 minutes at a moderate effort level, approximately 75 percent of your maximum heart rate.
Friday	Step 26-30 minutes at a moderate effort level, approximately 75 percent of your maximum heart rate.
Saturday	Skate 28 minutes using an interval training procedure: 5 minutes warm-up, 60 percent maximum heart rate 2 minutes lower-effort interval, 70 percent maximum heart rate 4 minutes higher-effort interval, 80 percent maximum heart rate 2 minutes lower-effort interval, 70 percent maximum heart rate 4 minutes higher-effort interval, 80 percent maximum heart rate 2 minutes lower-effort interval, 70 percent maximum heart rate 4 minutes higher-effort interval, 80 percent maximum heart rate 5 minutes cool-down, 60 percent maximum heart rate

Week Three

Monday	Cycle 26-30 minutes at a moderate effort level, approximately 75 percent of your maximum heart rate.
Wednesday	Step 26-30 minutes at a moderate effort level, approximately 75 percent of your maximum heart rate.
Friday	Cycle 26-30 minutes at a moderate effort level, approximately 75 percent of your maximum heart rate.

Saturday

Step 28 minutes using an interval training procedure:

5 minutes warm-up, 60 percent maximum heart rate
2 minutes lower-effort interval, 70 percent maximum heart rate
4 minutes higher-effort interval, 80 percent maximum heart rate
2 minutes lower-effort interval, 70 percent maximum heart rate
4 minutes higher-effort interval, 80 percent maximum heart rate
2 minutes lower-effort interval, 70 percent maximum heart rate
4 minutes higher-effort interval, 80 percent maximum heart rate
5 minutes cool-down, 60 percent maximum heart rate

Week Four

Monday

Skate 26-30 minutes at a moderate effort level, approximately 75 percent of your maximum heart rate.

Wednesday

Walk or jog 26-30 minutes at a moderate effort level, approximately 75 percent of your maximum heart rate.

Friday

Skate 26-30 minutes at a moderate effort level, approximately 75 percent of your maximum heart rate.

Saturday

Walk or jog 28 minutes using an interval training procedure:

5 minutes warm-up, 60 percent maximum heart rate
2 minutes lower-effort interval, 70 percent maximum heart rate
4 minutes higher-effort interval, 80 percent maximum heart rate
2 minutes lower-effort interval, 70 percent maximum heart rate
4 minutes higher-effort interval, 80 percent maximum heart rate
2 minutes lower-effort interval, 70 percent maximum heart rate
4 minutes higher-effort interval, 80 percent maximum heart rate
5 minutes cool-down, 60 percent maximum heart rate

* *If this equipment is not available, you may substitute similar endurance exercises.*

SUMMARY

The sample six-month endurance training program provides a framework for progressively developing higher levels of cardiovascular fitness. It starts with a month of less stressful recumbent cycling to begin getting you in shape. Treadmill walking, skating, and stepping give you variety and further conditioning over the next three months. After four months of aerobic cross-training at moderate effort levels, more challenging interval training begins. By the sixth month, the program involves four endurance exercise sessions a week, alternating more stressful and less stressful activities. Keep in mind that the monthly progressions are merely suggestions and that you may stay with any program as long as you desire.

Although you may substitute different aerobic activities and exercise procedures in the sample six-month training program, please use the following guidelines for safe and successful cardiovascular conditioning experiences.

- Warm up before and cool down after each workout.
- Train at a moderate effort level, between 60 and 80 percent of maximum heart rate.
- Progress in a gradual and systematic manner from one training session to the next.
- Use cross-training in a variety of aerobic activities to reduce the risk of overtraining injuries.
- Perform interval training to increase your exercise intensity without changing your workout time commitment.
- Maintain a regular exercise schedule, but do not hesitate to skip a training session if you are ill, injured, or fatigued.

CHAPTER 12

Fitness Program Design and Evaluation

Okay, you understand the training principles and procedures for developing muscular strength and cardiovascular endurance. But how do you put everything together into an integrated program of strength and endurance exercise?

TWO QUESTIONS

There are two major concerns related to a combination program of strength and endurance exercise. They are the arrangement of activities and the number of workouts a week.

Arrangement of Activities

The first question is, "How should you arrange the activities in a given training session?" Should you do the endurance exercise before the strength exercise or the strength exercise before the endurance exercise? Actually, the order of the activities has little effect on the training results, as long as you follow the recommended exercise guidelines. In one study, the participants did a high-effort Nautilus workout before a high-effort endurance workout and vice versa (1). The total strength train-

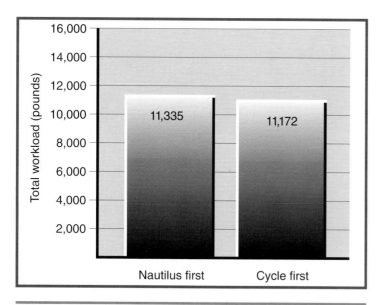

Fig. 12.1 Effects of activity order on strength performance during an 11-station Nautilus workout (8 subjects).

ing workloads performed were about the same regardless of the order of the activities (see figure 12.1).

Another study examined the effects of activity order on strength development over an eight-week training period (2). Half of the 43 subjects always performed the strength exercise before the endurance exercise, and the other half always did the endurance exercise before the strength exercise. Both training programs resulted in similar strength gains (see figure 12.2). So, feel free to choose your own activity order.

Endurance athletes should perform endurance exercise first, and strength athletes should do strength exercise first. But if your objective is overall physical fitness, this basic exercise procedure is recommended: Begin with a progressive warm-up for a smooth transition from rest to vigorous activity. Next, do your endurance exercise, followed by your strength exercise. Finally, gradually cool down to restore normal blood circulation and resting metabolism. This is also a good time for a few stretching exercises to finish your training session feeling loose and relaxed.

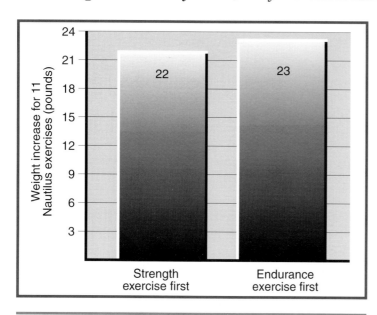

Fig. 12.2 Effects of activity order on strength gains during an eight-week program of strength and endurance exercise (43 subjects).

Number of Workouts

The second and more critical question is, "How many strength and endurance workouts should you do each week?" It is easy to overtrain when combining strength and endurance exercise. One study showed that a five-day-a-week program of strength and endurance training reduced overall benefits (3). The combined strength and endurance group

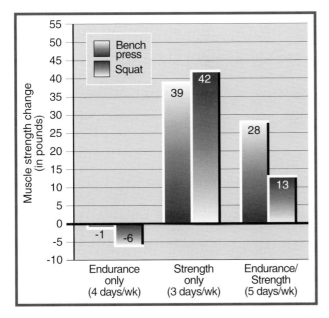

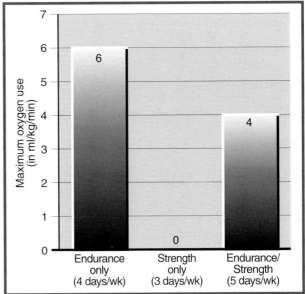

Fig. 12.3 Eight-week changes in muscle strength for three training groups (41 subjects), measuring the bench press and squat exercises.

Fig. 12.4 Eight-week changes in cardiovascular endurance for three training groups (41 subjects).

developed less strength than the strength-only group (see figure 12.3) and less endurance than the endurance-only group (see figure 12.4). Five days a week of combined strength and endurance training was apparently too much for achieving maximum gains in either muscular strength or cardiovascular endurance.

Fortunately, a similar study demonstrated excellent results from a three-day-a-week combination program (4). The combined strength and endurance group developed as much strength as the strength-only group (see figure 12.5) and almost as much endurance as the endurance-only group (see figure 12.6). So the three-day-a-week program of combined strength and endurance exercise effectively and efficiently achieved maximum gains in muscular strength and near-maximum gains in cardiovascular endurance.

Based on these results, a three-day-a-week combined strength and endurance program would be more beneficial. For example, you may train on Mondays, Wednesdays, and Fridays and rest the remainder of the week. If your emphasis is on cardiovascular conditioning, you may increase the number of aerobic workouts, but the extra training could limit your strength development. If your emphasis is on muscular conditioning, you may work harder but not more frequently because your muscles require about two days for strength building processes to be completed. If your goal is an injury-free exercise program that produces a high level of physical fitness, it's hard to beat a three-day-a-week combined strength and endurance program.

A combined program does not have to take an unreasonable amount of time. Both the sample strength training sessions given in chapter 6

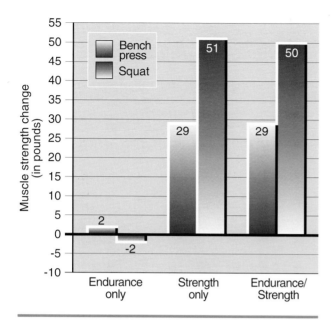

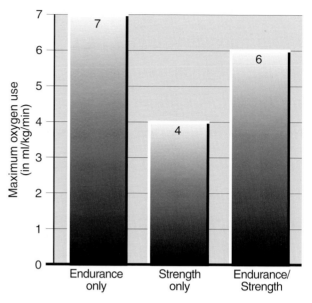

Fig. 12.5 Ten-week changes in muscle strength for three training groups (30 subjects, three days per week), measuring the bench press and squat exercises.

Fig. 12.6 Ten-week changes in cardiovascular endurance for three training groups (41 subjects) exercising three days per week.

and the sample endurance training sessions given in chapter 11 take about 25 to 30 minutes each.

Based on the programs described in chapters 6 and 11, program 12.1 shows a sample combination training program with approximate time segments for all of the exercise components. Although you may make periodic changes in your exercise program, the one-hour combined activity format is an effective and efficient approach for reaching high levels of muscular and cardiovascular fitness.

STRETCHING

While most of us agree that stretching exercises are useful for enhancing our joint flexibility and overall physical fitness, we do not always find time for this part of our exercise program. Because we try to do about 30 minutes of strength exercise and 30 minutes of endurance exercise each session, there is little room in a one-hour workout for stretching.

Although properly performed strength training alone improves joint flexibility, you still should do stretching exercises. The key muscle-joint structures that should be addressed in a stretching program include the following:

- Calf muscles, which cross the ankle and knee joints
- Hamstrings, which cross the knee and hip joints

PROGRAM 12.1

Sample strength and endurance training session with approximate time segments.

Time frame	General activity	Specific exercises
0-5 minutes	Warm-up (see chapter 11, month 5)	Easy cycling at 60% maximum heart rate
5-23 minutes	Endurance exercise (see chapter 11, month 5)	Interval cycling alternating 3 minutes at 70% maximum heart rate and 3 minutes at 80% maximum heart rate
23-28 minutes	Cool-down (see chapter 11, month 5)	Easy cycling at 60% maximum heart rate
30-58 minutes	Strength exercise (see chapter 6, month 5)	One set each of leg extension, seated leg curl, hip adductor, hip abductor, chest, super pullover, lateral raise, preacher curl, triceps extension, low back, rotary torso, 4-way neck, and chin-dip
58-63 minutes	Cool-down and stretching	Hamstrings stretch, low back stretch, shoulder stretch, calf stretch

- Low back muscles, which lie on both sides of the vertebral column
- Rotator cuff muscles, which surround the shoulder joints

Although some of these muscles are large and others are small, the basic stretching procedure is about the same. Gradually stretch the target muscle until it is comfortably lengthened, then hold that position for at least 30 seconds. This gentle approach reduces the risk of overstretching and maintains the stretched position long enough to experience positive muscle adaptations. If you have time, it may help to perform each stretch twice.

You may do stretching exercises while warming up or cooling down, or both. The cool-down is better for you for two reasons. First, your muscles are warmer and more stretchable after your workout. Second, stretching exercises serve as an excellent transition from activity to rest, helping you leave your training session feeling relaxed rather than tight.

THE "BIG FOUR" STRETCHING EXERCISES

Although you may include additional stretching exercises if you like, the "Big Four" sequence of stretches are ideal for developing flexibility. They are the step stretch, figure "4" stretch, letter "T" stretch, and doorway stretch. When performed properly, these stretches should enhance flexibility in your key muscle-joint structures.

Step Stretch

The step stretch targets the calf muscles in the lower leg. Because these muscles cross both your knee and ankle joints, keep your knee straight as you perform this exercise. Stand with your right foot fully on the step and your left foot half on and half off the step. Place one hand on the handrail or wall for balance. Gently shift your weight to your left foot and allow your left heel to slowly drop downward. As soon as your left calf muscles feel comfortably stretched, hold the position for at least 30 seconds. Change foot positions and repeat the same procedure for your right calf muscles (see figure 12.7).

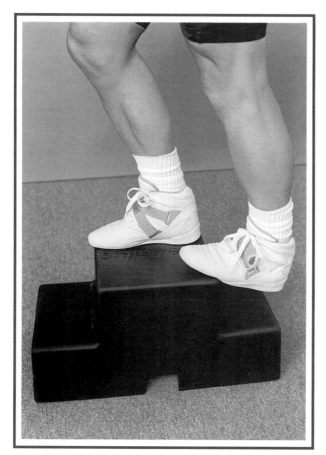

Fig. 12.7 The step stretch should be done one leg at a time for best results.

Figure "4" Stretch

This stretch resembles the "4" for which it is named. Although it actually addresses several muscles, you should feel the greatest stretch in the hamstrings at the back of the thighs (see figure 12.8). Begin by sitting on the floor with your left leg straight and your right leg bent at the knee so that your right foot touches your left thigh. Reach your left hand toward your left foot slowly, until your hamstrings feel comfortably stretched. At this point, grasp your foot, ankle, or lower leg and hold the stretched position for at least 30 seconds. Change leg positions and repeat the same procedure for your right hamstrings. You should also feel some stretching effects in your calf, hip, low back, and shoulder muscles as you do the figure "4" stretch.

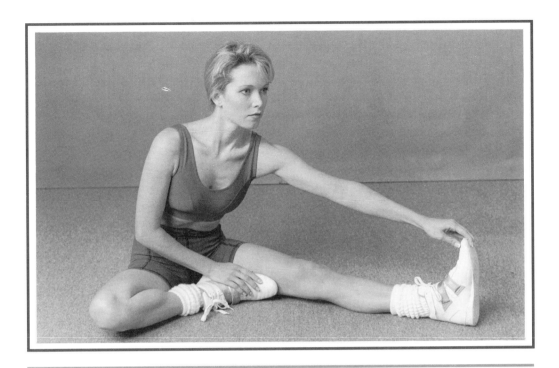

Fig. 12.8 The figure "4" stretch is ideal for safely stretching your hamstring muscles.

Letter "T" Stretch

As you may imagine, this stretch resembles the letter "T". It is designed to stretch the low back and hip muscles from a stable back position (see figure 12.9). Start by lying faceup on the floor with your arms straight out to the sides in a "T" position. Slowly lift your left leg upward, then

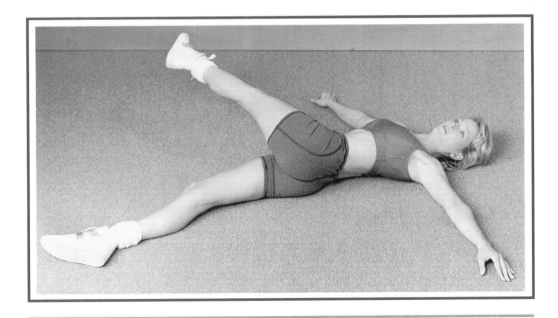

Fig. 12.9 The letter "T" stretch addresses both your low back and hip muscles.

cross it over so that your left foot is near (or touching) your right hand. Hold this comfortably stretched position for at least 30 seconds. Return your left leg to the starting position and repeat the same procedure with your right leg. Do your best to keep one leg straight as you carefully cross the other leg over your body.

Doorway Stretch

This two-part stretching exercise targets some of the shoulder rotator cuff muscles. But before beginning the doorway stretch, you may want to do some very slow arm circles to loosen up your shoulder joint. Part one of the doorway stretch begins by standing in a doorway with your right arm across your body and grasping the left door frame at about shoulder level. Gently turn your body to the right until your rear shoulder muscles feel comfortably stretched. Hold this position for at least 30 seconds. Part two begins by grasping the right door frame with your right arm at about shoulder level. Gently turn your body to the left until your front shoulder muscles feel comfortably stretched. Hold this position for a minimum of 30 seconds. Repeat these two stretches with your left arm.

Keep in mind that controlled, slow stretching is critical for safety and success. A lack of muscle tension and a relaxed sensation should characterize the stretching process. Always avoid trying too hard and stretching into the discomfort zone (see figure 12.10). The "Big Four" stretching sequence is a great way to conclude your exercise sessions, leaving you feeling invigorated rather than exhausted.

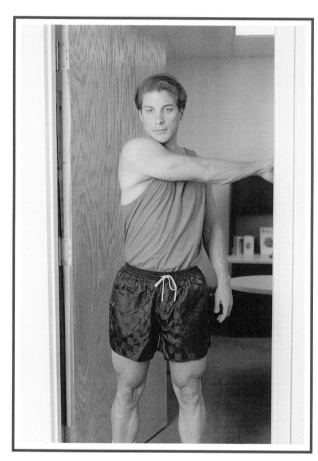

Fig. 12.10 The doorway stretch should be done gently and slowly.

EVALUATING YOUR PROGRESS

Your physical fitness program should be pleasant, satisfying, and rewarding. As a result of your exercise efforts, you should feel, function, and look better.

Still, many of us appreciate objective assessments of our progress as well as norms by which we can evaluate our personal fitness. As explained earlier in the book, four specific areas related to overall physical fitness are body composition, muscular strength, joint flexibility, and cardiovascular endurance. They are good areas to examine when judging your overall progress.

Body Composition

Body composition refers to your ratio of fat weight to lean weight and is usually reported as percent body fat. As discussed in chapter 2, men should be about 15 percent fat weight and 85 percent lean weight, while women should be about 20 percent fat weight and 80 percent lean weight. Your body composition can be assessed quite accurately at most fitness centers by means of skinfold calipers or bioelectrical impedance technology.

What if you are overweight but don't have access to body composition assessment equipment? You may still evaluate personal improvements in this area by taking periodic waist measurements. Stand "tall" and place a measuring tape around your waist just above your belt. At a normal rate of body composition improvement, you should see about a one-half-inch reduction in your waist measurement each month of training.

Muscular Strength

Muscular strength is related to your body weight and to your exercise program. That is, larger individuals are typically stronger than smaller individuals, and trained muscles are usually stronger than untrained muscles. For this reason, be sure to use strength assessments that adjust for body weight and address key muscle groups, such as the quadriceps.

Perhaps the best muscular strength assessment is the YMCA Leg Extension Test, based on data from over 900 men and women (5). Because the YMCA Leg Extension Test uses your 10-repetition maximum weight load, it is a safe strength assessment with a low risk of injury. And because it addresses the large and regularly used quadriceps, it is a practical test of muscular strength. Because the YMCA Leg Extension Test evaluates your strength relative to your body weight, it provides fair strength comparisons for men and women of various sizes.

If appropriate testing equipment is not available, you may evaluate your strength improvement by periodically comparing your exercise weight loads. Generally speaking, your exercise weight loads should increase about 45 percent during the first two months of training and about 15 percent during the next two months of training. After that, a 5 percent strength improvement every two months is excellent. For example, if you can leg press 100 pounds, you should be able to leg press about 145 pounds after two months of training, approximately 165 pounds after four months of training, and almost 175 pounds after six months of training.

YMCA Leg Extension Test

- Select a weight load on the Nautilus leg extension machine that is about 30 to 40 percent of your body weight.
- Perform 10 repetitions in the following manner:
  1. Lift the roller pad in two seconds to full knee extension.
  2. Hold the fully contracted position for one second.
  3. Lower the roller pad in four seconds until the weight stack lightly touches.
- If you complete 10 repetitions, rest two minutes, select a weight load that is 50 percent of your body weight, and perform 10 repetitions.
- Continue testing this way until you find the heaviest weight load that you can do for 10 repetitions.
- Divide this weight load by your body weight to determine your strength quotient.
- Locate your strength quotient in the appropriate strength-fitness classification described below.

Strength-quotient classifications		
Muscle strength	**Men**	**Women**
Low	49% body weight or below	39% body weight or below
Below average	50-59% body weight	40-49% body weight
Average	60-69% body weight	50-59% body weight
Above average	70-79% body weight	60-69% body weight
High	80% body weight or above	70% body weight or above

According to this assessment technique, a 120-pound woman who performs 10 leg extensions with 60 pounds has a strength quotient of 50 percent—average strength in her quadriceps.

Joint Flexibility

Joint flexibility refers to the movement range of a given joint structure. It is highly specific and may vary considerably from joint to joint. Because poor hip-trunk flexibility may be related to low back problems, this is the

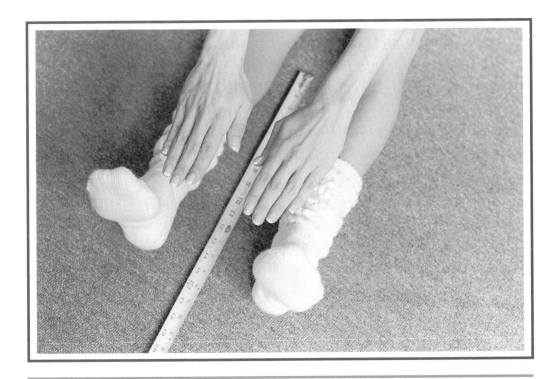

Fig. 12.11   You can easily monitor improvement in your hip-trunk flexibility.

area most frequently evaluated in flexibility tests. If you have good hip-trunk flexibility you should be able to touch your toes without bending your knees. To avoid back strain, do this assessment in a sitting—rather than a standing—position.

To evaluate your hip-trunk flexibility, sit on the floor with a yardstick between your legs, lining up the 15-inch mark with your heels (see figure 12.11). With your knees straight, reach forward as far as possible without straining. If you can touch the 15-inch mark, you are reasonably flexible in the hip-trunk area. If you cannot stretch this far, an inch a month increase is an excellent rate of improvement. Although you may be able to reach beyond your toes, don't try to develop extreme flexibility, as excessive joint mobility may increase your risk of injury.

Cardiovascular Endurance

Cardiovascular endurance is primarily a measure of your ability to perform aerobic activity. Most fitness centers offer cardiovascular endurance assessments using cycle, treadmill, or step tests.

If you do not have access to supervised evaluation techniques, you may measure your cardiovascular progress in less formal ways. For a general assessment, periodically monitor your resting heart rate. Your resting heart rate typically slows down as your cardiovascular condition improves, so a progressive reduction in your resting heart rate indicates an effective training program.

Another assessment procedure is to periodically compare your training heart rates at a given exercise level. As your cardiovascular fitness increases, your training heart rate at the same work level should decrease. For example, during your first month of training, treadmill walking at three miles an hour may raise your heart rate to 140 beats a minute. During your second month of training, this same workout may elevate your heart rate to only 132 beats a minute, while during your third month of training, only to 124 heart beats a minute.

These assessment techniques may provide more objective information about your fitness development. The most revealing feature of a successful exercise program, however, is your training regularity. Without question, the critical factor in reaching and maintaining a high level of physical fitness is your training consistency. Regular training sessions with gradual improvement give more overall benefits than an occasional outstanding workout.

SUMMARY

A combination strength and endurance training program effectively improves both muscular and cardiovascular fitness. For best overall results, you should train three days a week and rest between exercise sessions. This encourages fitness development, giving your body time to adapt to physical changes between workouts and reducing your risk of injury. Although the activity order is a matter of personal preference, be sure to warm up before and cool down after each training session.

Periodically check your fitness progress with formal or informal assessment techniques. A well-designed exercise program should produce consistent improvements in your body composition, muscular strength, joint flexibility, and cardiovascular endurance. But the most important indicator of a physically productive and personally satisfying exercise program is your training regularity. You should look forward to each workout as a challenging and rewarding experience that is an essential part of your normal lifestyle.

CHAPTER 13

Advanced Training Programs

Congratulations! You are now ready for more advanced training. At this point, you may be working hard but making few fitness gains. As you achieve higher levels of fitness, your rate of improvement gradually slows down, and you eventually reach a training plateau. Although lack of progress may be discouraging, it is simply a sign that you should change your exercise program. Of course, everyone has different genetic potential for physical development, so you should approach advanced training in a sensible manner.

Should you do more work to further increase your muscular strength and cardiovascular endurance? Not necessarily. While more sets of strength exercise and longer periods of endurance exercise may be effective, this training approach poses two problems for most people.

First, more exercise sets and longer endurance sessions increase the training time, which is typically a limiting factor. Second, increasing the amount of exercise may lead to overtraining, fatigue, and injury—all of which are undesirable.

A more practical approach for overcoming fitness plateaus is to increase the exercise intensity without significantly increasing the exercise duration. There are several effective and efficient methods for moving into an advanced strength training program.

ADVANCED STRENGTH TRAINING

After a certain period of training, your muscles become less responsive to the regular workout routine, and a new exercise program is in order.

Overcoming Strength Training Plateaus

The three best approaches are to choose new exercises, change your training program, and increase your training intensity.

Choose New Exercises

Our first recommendation is to choose new training exercises. For example, if you are not progressing in the 10° chest exercise, substitute the 50° chest exercise. The slightly different movement pattern still targets the pectoralis major, but activates different muscle fibers and produces a new stimulus for strength development.

Periodically changing your training exercises may be the best way to prevent boredom and strength plateaus. You should stay, however, with a given exercise long enough to maximize your muscle response. Spend at least one month on each exercise to allow your muscles to adapt to the new training stimulus.

Change Training Program

In addition to choosing new training exercises, you should systematically vary your workout procedures. This is called *periodization* and involves changing the resistance and number of repetitions you use. For example, during month one you may complete 12 to 16 repetitions with lighter than normal resistance. During month two, you may do 8 to 12 repetitions with your normal weight loads. And during month three, you may perform 4 to 8 repetitions with heavier than normal resistance.

Another advantage of periodically changing your resistance-repetitions relationship is the use of different muscle fibers to stimulate further strength development. Just be sure to give each training program enough time to be effective. For continuity, don't change your strength workout more often than every four weeks.

Increase Training Intensity

You may choose to perform additional exercise sets to increase your training effort. Because performing more work requires more time and energy, you should increase the number of training sets gradually. If at present you are doing one set of each exercise, spend at least a month performing two sets of each exercise. If this proves successful, you may progress to three sets an exercise. Just be alert for signs of overtraining and schedule sufficient recovery time between workouts.

Because of the additional time needed for multiple-set training, many people do advanced strength training using a split routine in which they train certain muscle groups on certain days. For example, on Mondays and Thursdays, they may do exercises for their chests, shoulders, and triceps. On Tuesdays and Fridays, they may perform exercises for their backs and biceps. On Wednesdays and Saturdays they may do exercises for their legs, midsections, and necks. This way, they work each major muscle group twice a week but avoid lengthy training sessions. Of course, this requires a total of six training days a week, which may be impractical for many people.

Is it possible to increase your training intensity without adding workout time or exercise sessions? Yes. This is referred to as high-intensity training. As explained in chapter 3, three of the most effective high-intensity techniques are breakdown training, assisted training, and slow training. Prestretching can help you increase resistance. These high-intensity training techniques place greater demands on the target muscles, but require more tissue recovery and building time. For best results, you should perform high-intensity training no more than once or twice a week.

Breakdown Training. Breakdown training begins with a standard set of 8 to 12 repetitions. At the point of muscle fatigue, you lower the resistance enough to perform 2 to 4 additional repetitions. You typically must reduce the starting weight load 10 to 20 percent.

Assisted Training. Assisted training is similar to breakdown training in principle, but different in practice. Once again, you begin with a standard set of 8 to 12 repetitions. When you reach muscle fatigue, a trainer assists you with the lifting phase of 2 to 4 additional repetitions.

Slow Training. Instead of increasing the number of repetitions in each set, slow training increases the time each repetition takes. Four to 6 slow repetitions take about the same time as 8 to 12 normal repetitions, but the slower movement speed reduces momentum and increases muscle tension. You may do slow training with a positive emphasis (10 seconds up and 4 seconds down) or a negative emphasis (4 seconds up and 10 seconds down).

Prestretching. One method of using slightly higher resistance than would otherwise be possible is prestretching. Prestretching takes advantage of the "stretch reflex," which we have all experienced. For example, you don't simply jump from a flat-footed stance or move your hand forward to throw. Rather, you crouch quickly and then launch yourself, or you stretch your arm backwards before you throw. This "prestretching" increases your power in the positive movement which follows. In the same way, if you are doing, for example, a leg press exercise, when you reach the end of the movement range, allow the weight to quickly stretch your muscles a fraction of an inch further than you would normally go before resuming the positive lifting action at the normal speed. This produces the stretch reflex that allows you to begin your next repetition with slightly more force. Always prestretch with control, and avoid this technique on neck or low back exercises. Be sure you are in excellent shape before attempting it.

Research Results

A recent study compared the effects of different high-intensity training techniques on strength plateaus (1). The subjects performed breakdown training on three exercises, assisted training on three exercises, positive-emphasis slow training on three exercises, and negative-emphasis slow training on three exercises. They also did two exercises in the standard way, but under the supervision of a personal trainer who emphasized proper exercise technique. All of the training methods produced significant improvements in muscle strength, including the supervised standard training (see figure 13.1). Apparently, working with an instructor encourages better training technique and greater exercise effort. Each of the high-intensity techniques, however, produced even greater strength gains.

You should experiment with different high-intensity training methods to determine which techniques work best for you. Perhaps the most attractive feature of high-intensity training is that breakdown and assisted techniques take only a few extra seconds a set, while slow training takes no more time than standard training.

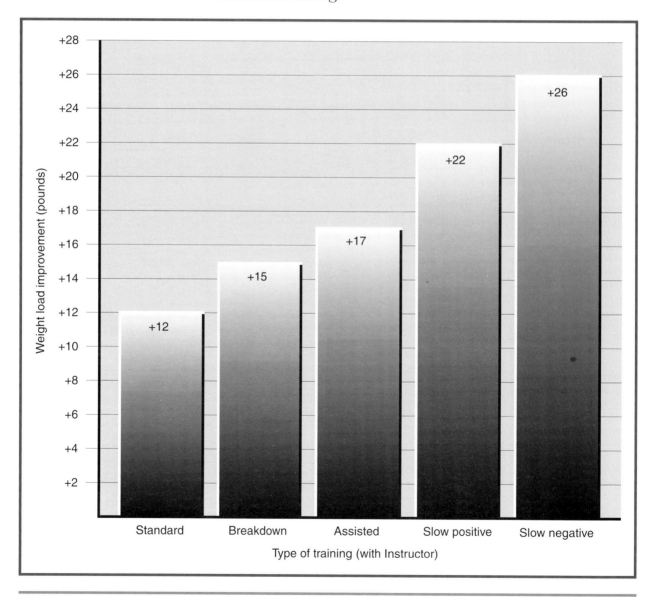

Fig. 13.1 Strength improvements for previously plateaued individuals after six weeks of supervised training using different exercise techniques (22 subjects).

Advanced strength training requires a good balance between your work effort and your recovery period. Too little stimulus or too much rest results in underdevelopment, while too much stimulus or too little rest

PROGRAM 13.1

Sample high-intensity strength training program for advanced exercisers.

Exercise	Procedure
Leg extension:	8-12 repetitions to fatigue, followed immediately by 2-4 assisted repetitions
Leg curl:	8-12 repetitions to fatigue, followed immediately by 2-4 assisted repetions
Leg press:	8-12 repetitions to fatigue
Chest cross:	8-12 repetitions to fatigue, followed immediately by chest press exercise
Chest press:	6-10 repetitions to fatigue—immediately following chest cross exercise
Super pullover:	8-12 repetitions to fatigue, followed immediately by compound row exercise
Compound row:	6-10 repetitions to fatigue—immediately following super-pullover exercise
Lateral raise:	4-6 repetitions at very slow speed, lifting in 10 seconds and lowering in 4 seconds
Preacher curl:	8-12 repetitions to fatigue, followed immediately by 2-4 breakdown repetitions with 10 pounds less resistance
Triceps extension:	8-12 repetitions to fatigue, followed immediately by 2-4 breakdown repetitions with 10 pounds less resistance
Low back:	8-12 repetitions to fatigue
Abdominal:	8-12 repetitions to fatigue
Neck extension:	8-12 repetitions to fatigue
Neck flexion:	8-12 repetitions to fatigue

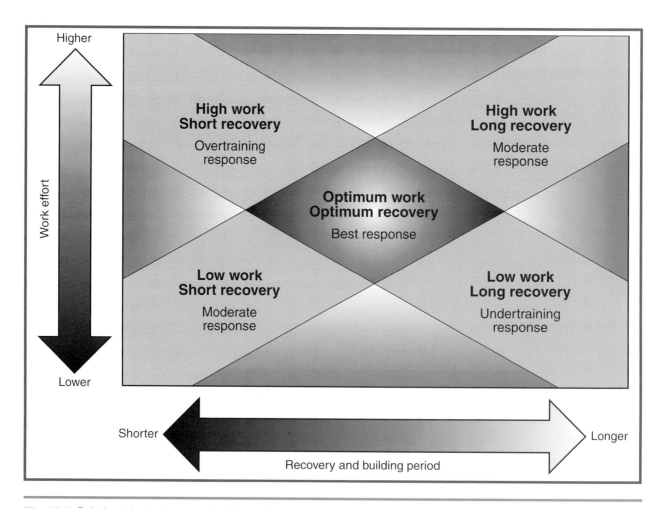

Fig. 13.2 Relationships between work effort and recovery period.

results in overtraining. For best results, let the sample high-intensity workout shown in program 13.1 serve as a guide for your advanced training sessions, keeping your work effort and recovery period in the shaded area shown in figure 13.2.

ADVANCED ENDURANCE TRAINING

In contrast to strength training, increasing the exercise duration may enhance your endurance development. Just be careful to increase the training time gradually and avoid overtraining. Most authorities recommend the 10 percent rule for increasing your endurance exercise sessions. That is, after the initial conditioning stage (about one month), you should add only 10 percent more training time each week. For example, if at present you are cycling for 30 minutes a session, you should not increase the training time more than three minutes a session each week.

Change Training Activities

Like strength training, changing the exercise activities may benefit you both physiologically and psychologically. Different endurance activities involve different muscles, requiring a different cardiovascular response. For example, if you are not advancing in your cycling exercise, switch to another aerobic activity, such as walking, jogging, skating, or stepping. If you prefer doing a single activity each workout, stay with the new exercise at least one month to allow your body to adapt to the demands of that activity.

You may also change exercises within a given endurance training session as long as you maintain reasonable workout consistency. Cross-training enables you to attain a high cardiovascular effort while working different muscle groups. For example, a 30-minute cross-training session could be divided into 10 minutes of stepping, 10 minutes of recumbent cycling, and 10 minutes of skating. In this way, you emphasize the front thigh muscles, then the rear thigh muscles, then the inner and outer thigh muscles. Of course, your heart is pumping hard throughout every phase of the cross-training workout. Program 13.2 shows a sample cross-training session for advanced endurance training.

PROGRAM 13.2

Sample cross-training program for advanced endurance exercisers.

Time (minutes)	Activity	Percent maximum heart rate
4	Warm-up cycling	
8	Cycling	75
8	Skating	75
8	Treadmill jogging	75
4	Cool-down treadmill walking	
Total workout time = 32 minutes		

Increase Training Demands

Although steady pace exercise offers a productive approach to endurance development, your cardiovascular system may eventually become accustomed to the same training effort. Interval training is an effective means for increasing the workout demands without increasing the exercise duration.

Consider a 32-minute cycling session that includes a 4-minute warm-up, a 4-minute cool-down, and 24 minutes of moderate-effort endurance training (about 75 percent of maximum heart rate). Now divide the 24-minute conditioning session into six intervals of 4 minutes each. Perform the first, third, and fifth interval at a higher effort level (about 85 percent of maximum heart rate) and do the second, fourth, and sixth interval at a lower effort level (about 65 percent of maximum heart rate). Although the average heart rate response is similar to steady pace exercise, this workout requires a harder training effort and conditions you better.

You may redesign your interval training program in a variety of ways to ensure progressive cardiovascular development. For example, you may gradually increase the length of the higher-effort intervals, while gradually decreasing the length of the lower-effort intervals. As your cardiovascular fitness improves, you can increase your training level for both the higher-effort and lower-effort intervals. The key to successful interval training is doing three or more challenging rounds of aerobic exercise during each endurance workout. Program 13.3 shows a sample interval training session for advanced endurance training.

PROGRAM 13.3

Sample interval training program for advanced exercisers.

35-minute recumbent cycling workout

Time (minutes)	Activity	Percent maximum heart rate
4	Warm-up cycling	60
6	Higher-effort cycling interval	80
3	Lower-effort cycling interval	70
6	Higher-effort cycling interval	80
3	Lower-effort cycling interval	70
6	Higher-effort cycling interval	80
3	Lower-effort cycling interval	70
4	Cool-down cycling	60

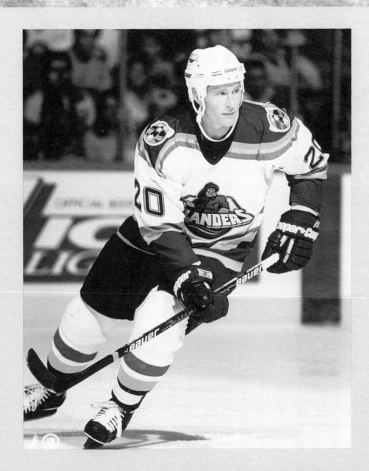

Bob Sweeney began his long hockey career at Acton-Boxboro High School. During the 1981-1982 season, he lead eastern Massachusetts in scoring with 90 points. In 1982, he was named to the *Boston Globes*'s all scholastic team. His #7 is the only retired jersey hanging in Acton-Boxboro High School's rafters.

Although drafted in the sixth round in 1982, Bob chose to attend Boston College, where he earned a BA in finance. During his four years at BC, he was a member of the Eagles hockey team. He was the Bean Pot MVP in 1983 and was named 2nd-team All-American in 1985. His BC teams had a four-year string of NCAA Tournament bids.

After graduation in 1986, he joined the Boston Bruins, scoring 64 goals and 103 assists during his six years there. In 1991, he was traded to the Buffalo Sabres and was instrumental in upsetting the Bruins in the 1993 playoffs. He spent three years with the Sabres before moving on to the NY Islanders for a year. He is currently a member of the Calgary Flames.

Bob combines a basic strength training program with regular endurance exercise, particularly running and cycling. His running workouts often involve interval training to improve both performance power and cardiovascular fitness. His strength workouts are typically hard and brief, with an emphasis on all of the major muscle groups. This type of training provides excellent results and leaves plenty of time for practicing hockey.

SUMMARY

At some point in your exercise program you will experience a fitness plateau. If you are satisfied with your current physical condition, you need not train harder or progress further. If you like your standard exercise routine, simply continue your training program and you will maintain your present fitness level. If you prefer variety, then you should periodically change your exercises and your training program. In any case, you need not do advanced workouts unless you want to.

If your progress levels off before you reach your fitness goals, however, advanced training procedures should be helpful. Just remember that everyone has different genetic potential for physical performance, so advanced training must be approached sensibly.

Strength plateaus respond well to different training exercises and varied training programs and procedures. Increasing the number of training sets may be productive, but you must be careful to avoid overtraining. A more efficient advanced training approach is to increase the exercise intensity, which may be done by adding repetitions to each exercise set (breakdown or assisted training), by adding time to each exercise repetition (slow training), or by the cautious use of prestretching. High-intensity training programs are effective for overcoming strength plateaus and increasing your muscular fitness. But because of the greater demands and longer recovery period, you should limit high-intensity training to one or two exercise sessions a week.

To overcome endurance plateaus, you may change the exercise activity or do cross-training. Like strength training, however, further fitness improvements may require more demanding exercise sessions. Interval training is an excellent way to increase the exercise effort without lengthening the exercise time. Training with higher- and lower-effort intervals creates a more challenging exercise program and enhances your cardiovascular fitness. Just be sure to alternate your interval workouts with steady pace sessions to maintain a balanced training program.

Free-Weight Exercises

Free weights are economical tools that can provide progressive resistance for most of the major muscle groups. Their compactness make them a popular choice for at-home strength training.

Using free weights properly requires careful instruction and safety awareness. Because some barbell exercises have a high injury risk, these should be performed only with assistance from a spotter. Practice safe strength training by seeking proper instruction before you exercise with free weights.

The exercises presented here cover most of the major muscle categories used for the strength training equipment:

1. Leg exercises
2. Chest exercises
3. Upper back exercises
4. Shoulder exercises
5. Arm exercises
6. Midsection exercises

The precautions given in chapter 5 for exercise performance apply especially to free-weight exercises. When you perform your strength exercises using free weights, follow the training tips carefully.

Barbell Squat

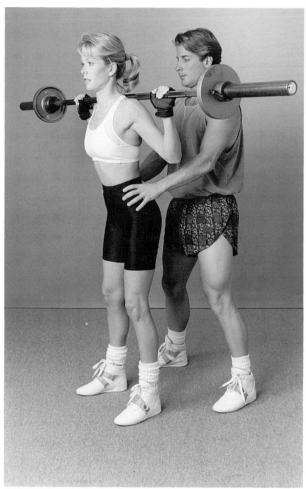

a

Joint Action
Hip extension and knee extension

Prime Mover Muscles
Hamstrings, gluteals, and quadriceps

Movement Path
Linear

Exercise Technique
- Stand with feet slightly wider than shoulder width apart.
- Lift barbell from supports, with bar resting across upper back, bracing with hands.
- Slowly lower body until thighs are about parallel to the floor, then return to standing position.

Technique Tips
- Keep back and head erect throughout the exercise.
- Keep feet flat on the floor.
- For safety's sake never perform barbell squats without a spotter.
- Because free weights do not provide variable resistance, more than one set may be necessary.

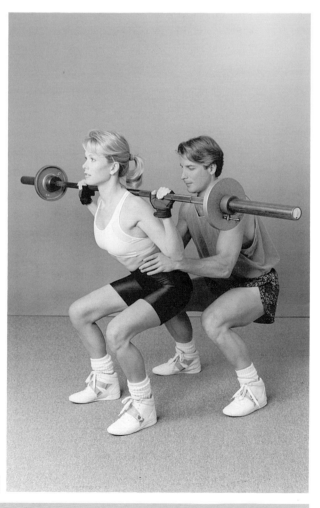

b

Barbell Bench Press

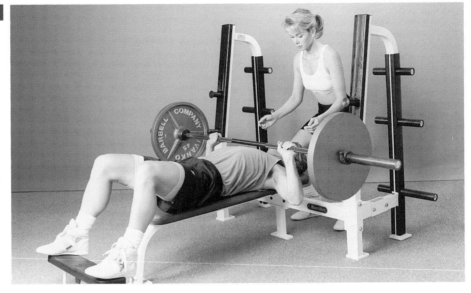

a

Joint Action
Shoulder horizontal flexion and elbow extension

Prime Mover Muscles
Pectoralis major, anterior deltoid, and triceps

Movement Path
Linear

Exercise Technique
- Lie on bench with head below barbell.
- Grasp barbell slightly wider than shoulder width and lift from supports.
- Slowly lower barbell to chest, press upward to starting position, and repeat.

Technique Tips
- Keep head and hips on bench.
- Keep feet on floor or footrest.
- Do not arch the back or bounce the barbell off the chest. For safety's sake, never perform barbell bench presses without a spotter.
- Because free weights do not provide variable resistance, more than one set may be necessary.

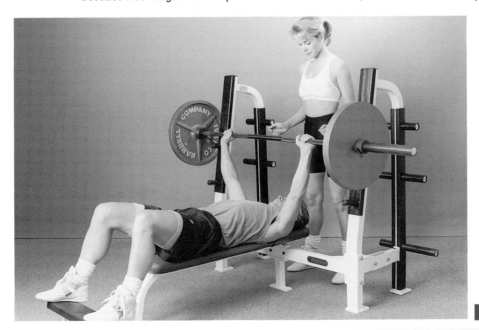

b

Dumbbell Bent Row

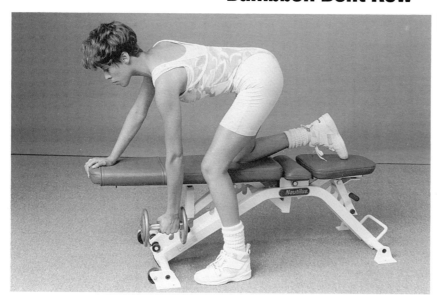

a

Joint Action
Shoulder extension and elbow flexion

Prime Mover Muscles
Latissimus dorsi, teres major, biceps

Movement Path
Linear

Exercise Technique
- Place right knee and right hand on bench so that back is about parallel to the floor.
- Grasp dumbbell with left hand and pull to chest.
- Lower dumbbell slowly and repeat.
- Repeat exercise with right hand.

Technique Tips
- Maintain neutral head position.
- Keep elbow relatively close to body during lifting and lowering movements.
- Because free weights do not provide variable resistance, more than one set may be necessary.

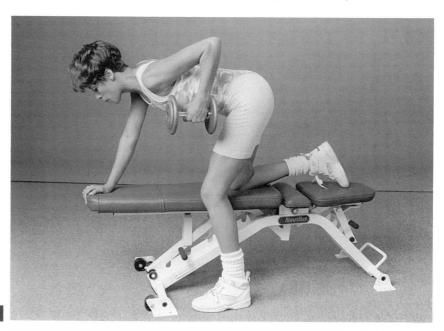

b

Dumbbell Overhead Press

a

Joint Action
Shoulder abduction and elbow extension

Prime Mover Muscles
Deltoids and triceps

Movement Path
Linear

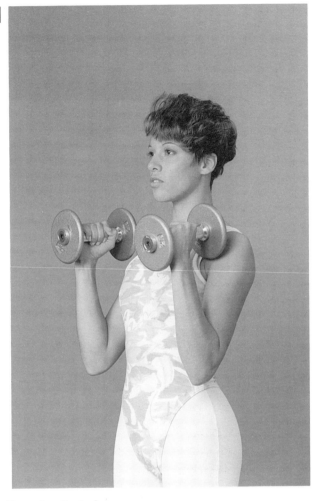

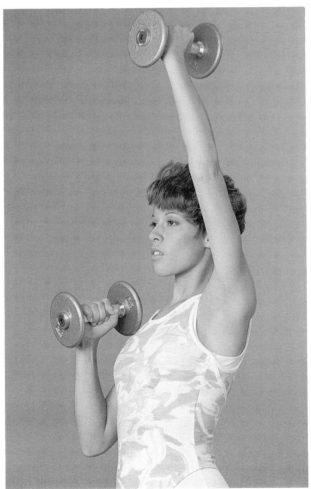

Exercise Technique
- Stand with feet about shoulder width apart and lift dumbells to shoulders.
- Press the left dumbbell overhead and lower slowly back to shoulder.
- Press the right dumbbell overhead and lower slowly back to shoulder.
- Repeat alternating pressing movements.

Technique Tips
- Keep back and head erect throughout the exercise.
- Alternate left and right arm action.
- Because free weights do not provide variable resistance, more than one set may be necessary.

b

Dumbbell Biceps Curl

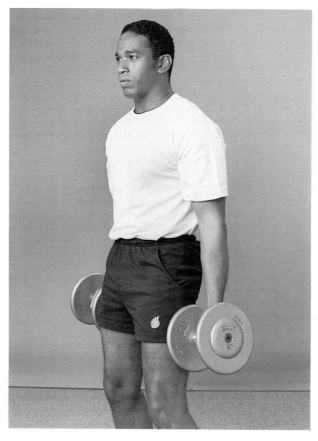

a

Joint Action
Elbow flexion

Prime Mover Muscles
Biceps

Movement Path
Rotary

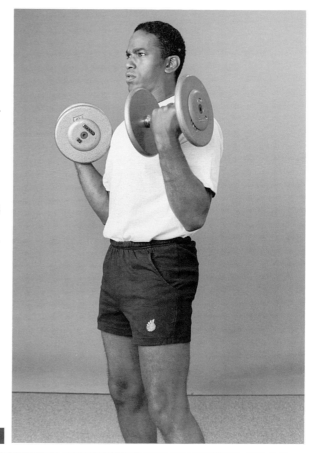

Exercise Technique
- Stand with feet about shoulder width apart, holding dumbbells at thighs.
- Curl dumbbells to shoulders.
- Return slowly to starting position and repeat.

Technique Tips
- Keep back and head erect and elbows against sides throughout the exercise.
- Because free weights do not provide variable resistance, more than one set may be necessary.

b

Dumbbell Triceps Kickback

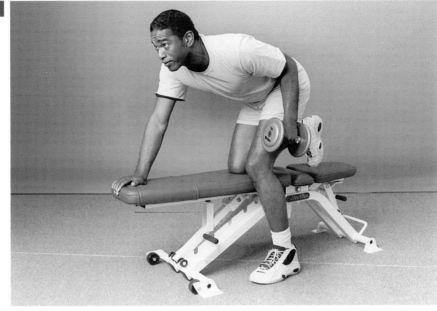

Joint Action
Elbow extension

Prime Mover Muscles
Triceps

Movement Path
Rotary

Exercise Technique
- Place right knee and right hand on bench so that back is about parallel to floor.
- Grasp dumbbell with left hand and place elbow against side, with forearm perpendicular to floor.
- Extend elbow backward until forearm is parallel to floor.
- Return slowly to starting position and repeat.
- Repeat exercise with right hand.

Technique Tips
- Maintain neutral head position.
- Keep elbow against side during lifting and lowering movements.
- Because free weights do not provide variable resistance, more than one set may be necessary.

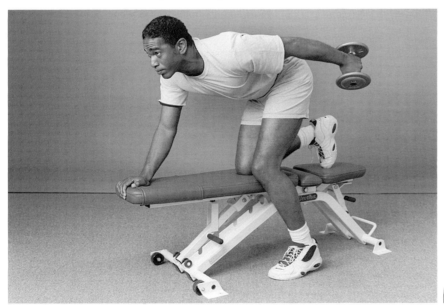

Trunk Curl

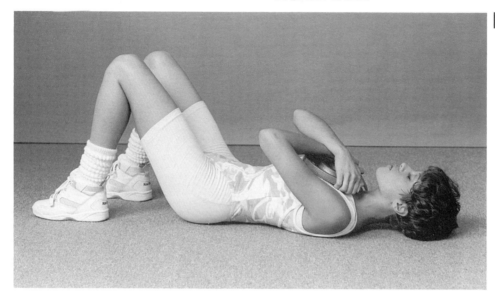

a

Joint Action
Trunk flexion

Prime Mover Muscles
Rectus abdominis

Movement Path
Rotary

Exercise Technique
- Lie on mat with knees bent and holding a 50-10 pound barbell plate on your chest.
- Slowly curl head and shoulders off the mat and press lower back into the mat.
- If you wish to decrease resistance, remove the plate and cup hands loosely around ears.
- Return slowly to starting position and repeat.

Technique Tips
- Maintain neutral head position.
- Because body weight exercises do not provide variable resistance, more than one set may be necessary.

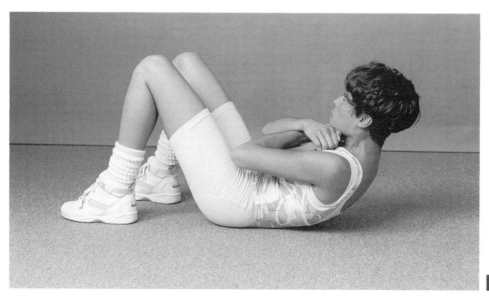

b

Choosing Your Fitness Facility

What should you look for when selecting the right fitness facility? If you are an experienced exerciser who needs little instruction and supervision, you should feel comfortable in most well-equipped and well-maintained exercise centers. If you are a beginner, however, you should train in a structured fitness facility that offers qualified instructors and strict exercise guidelines.

The South Shore YMCA Fitness Center (four full lines of Nautilus machines), which emphasizes member education and training, has experienced a high growth and retention rate over the past 12 years. In fact, this facility has been featured in numerous fitness magazines, and in 1995 was ranked the best buy in the exercise industry (1). As you search for a training facility, consider some of the management features that have helped our members achieve successful exercise experiences.

Member Orientation

Facilities that stress participant instruction usually provide orientation sessions for new members. Before our members begin training, they view a 25-minute video on exercise principles and procedures, complete a medical history form, and ask questions about their training program. They also receive an exercise manual and article reprints on relevant fitness topics. Our fitness directors conduct member orientation sessions twice each day.

Member Training

After completing the orientation session, new members sign up for the first of several one-on-one training sessions with one of our fitness instructors. We believe that quality instruction is the key to a positive and productive exercise program. Fitness centers with proper priorities have qualified instructional staff on duty at all times both to teach new members as well as to assist experienced members. Member training should be an ongoing process that ensures good exercise technique, enabling members to systematically progress to higher fitness levels.

Member Service

Member service may mean different things to different people. To us, it means a spacious facility with enough equipment for all of the members. It also means providing the best equipment and keeping it in perfect working order. Caring fitness centers have preventive maintenance programs that include periodic equipment tune-ups and daily cleaning of the exercise machines.

Concerned exercise centers have guidelines for using the equipment and for sharing the facility with other members. For example, ask if the club requires controlled movement speeds on the strength machines and see if spray bottles and towels are provided to clean the equipment upholstery after each use.

SUMMARY

When choosing a fitness facility, look for one where management shares their training philosophy, policies, and procedures up-front. Although there is no training center that is perfect for everyone, most adults appreciate a fitness facility that provides orientation, training, and service. They like a no-nonsense training environment, in which members use proper exercise technique, clean their machines after use, and progress through the equipment circuit in an orderly manner.

Two reasons many people avoid exercise facilities are lack of time and lack of confidence. Training centers that provide efficient exercise procedures and professional fitness instructors solve both of these problems. Do your best to find a well-managed, well-staffed, and well-equipped exercise center that facilitates your personal fitness improvement.

Fitness Dictionary

Anaerobic Exercise   High-intensity exercise that can be performed at a relatively high energy level for a relatively brief period of time (less than 90 seconds).

Antagonist Muscle   The muscle opposite the prime mover muscle that lengthens as the prime mover muscle shortens. For example, the biceps and triceps are antagonist muscles.

Atrophy   A decrease in muscle tissue that results from injury, lack of strength exercise, or the aging process.

Body Composition   The percentage of your body weight that is fat as opposed to lean tissue, such as muscle and bone. Males should be about 15 percent body fat and females should be about 20 percent body fat.

Cardiovascular Endurance   The capacity to perform low- to moderate-intensity exercise (cycling, walking, jogging, skating, stepping, etc.) for relatively long periods of time.

Circuit Strength Training   A strength training program in which you move quickly from exercise to exercise, usually in order from larger to smaller muscle groups (legs, torso, arms, midsection, neck).

Concentric Contraction   The target muscle shortens and produces enough force to lift the resistance. This is also called a positive contraction.

Direct Resistance Exercise   Exercise in which the resistance force is applied directly to the body part (e.g., upper arm) where the target muscle (e.g., deltoid) attaches. This assists in isolating the target muscle.

Dynamic Constant Resistance Exercise   Exercise in which the resistance force remains the same throughout the movement range.

Dynamic Variable Resistance Exercise   Exercise in which the resistance force changes in proportion to your muscle force throughout the movement range.

Eccentric Contraction   The target muscle lengthens and produces enough force to slowly lower the resistance. This is also called a negative contraction.

Fast-Twitch Muscle Fibers   The type of muscle fibers that produce higher levels of force for shorter periods of time.

Fitness Plateau A period without improvement in your exercise performance, indicating a need to change some aspect of your training program.

Full Movement Range Exercising the target muscle through a complete joint action, from the fully stretched to the fully contracted positions.

Hypertrophy An increase in muscle tissue that results from progressive strength exercise.

Interval Training Alternately performing higher-effort and lower-effort exercise segments throughout an endurance training session.

Maximum Heart Rate The fastest rate your heart will beat during maximum effort exercise. You can estimate your maximum heart rate by subtracting your age from 220.

Motor Unit All of the muscle fibers activated by a given motor nerve. Slow-twitch motor units typically have about 100 slow-twitch muscle fibers, and fast-twitch motor units typically have about 500 fast-twitch muscle fibers.

Muscle Balance Training all of your major muscle groups to attain balanced strength development and reduced risk of injuries.

Muscle Fatigue The point when the target muscles can no longer lift the resistance. Muscle fatigue may be related to the accumulation of lactic acid associated with high-effort anaerobic exercise.

Muscle Fiber The actual muscle cell that contracts upon stimulus to produce the force for movement.

Muscle Isolation Targeting a specific muscle (or muscle group) by using rotary movement and direct resistance exercise.

Muscle Length The length of the muscle relative to its attachments. Long muscles have short tendon attachments and a greater potential for increasing size and strength.

Muscular Endurance The capacity to perform high-intensity exercise (chin-ups, bar-dips, leg extensions, leg curls, etc.) for a relatively high number of repetitions.

Muscular Strength The capacity to perform high-intensity exercise with near-maximum resistance. Muscular strength is typically assessed by the heaviest resistance you can lift for 1 to 10 repetitions.

Overtraining Performing too much exercise to permit full recovery and tissue building between successive training sessions.

Perceived Exertion Level Your subjective rating of the exercise effort. Typically evaluated by your ability to talk during aerobic exercise.

Periodization Periodic and systematic variations in your strength training program.

Power   A measure of work output, power is the product of muscle force and movement speed.

Prime Mover Muscle   The muscle that contracts to produce the desired movement. For example, the triceps are the prime mover muscles for elbow extension exercises.

Progressive Resistance Exercise   An exercise program that permits gradual increases in resistance as the muscles become stronger. Add 5 percent more resistance when you can complete 12 repetitions.

Recovery Time   The rest period between training sessions during which the muscles build to higher strength levels.

Repetitions   The number of times you lift and lower the training resistance without resting. Performing 8 to 12 repetitions of each exercise is recommended.

Rotary Movement Exercise   Exercise in which the movement path is circular, around the joint axis of rotation. This assists in isolating the target muscle.

Set   The number of times you perform repetitions of a given exercise. For example, performing 10 leg extensions, resting one minute, and performing 10 more leg extensions equals two sets of 10 repetitions each.

Slow-Twitch Muscle Fibers   The type of muscle fibers that produce lower levels of force for longer periods of time.

Stabilizer Muscles   Muscles that stabilize the non-exercising joints of the body to facilitate desired movements in the target joints and muscles. For example, the low back and abdominal muscles stabilize your torso during the performance of neck flexion and extension exercises.

Steady Pace Training   Exercising at the same effort level throughout an endurance training session.

Training Duration   The time required to perform a set of strength exercises (set duration) or to complete your strength or endurance workout (session duration).

Training Frequency   The number of strength training or endurance training sessions per week.

Training Intensity   The effort level required to perform a given exercise. High-intensity training refers to higher-effort exercise that can be maintained for a relatively short duration. Low-intensity training refers to lower-effort exercise that can be maintained for a relatively long duration.

Variable Resistance Exercise   Exercise that automatically changes the resistance throughout the movement range. Ideally, the resistance should decrease proportionately in positions of lower muscle force and increase proportionately in positions of higher muscle force.

References

Chapter 1

1. Centers for Disease Control. 1989. Physical activity, physical fitness, and health: Time to act. *JAMA* 262: 2437.

2. Campbell, W., and M. Crim, V. Young, and W. Evans. 1994. Increased energy requirements and changes in body composition with resistance training in older adults. *American Journal of Clinical Nutrition* 60: 167-175.

3. Westcott, W. 1995. *Strength fitness: Physiological principles and training techniques.* 4th Ed. Dubuque, IA: Brown and Benchmark.

4. Frontera, W., C. Meredith, K. O'Reilly et al. 1988. Strength conditioning in older men: Skeletal muscle hypertrophy and improved function. *Journal of Applied Physiology* 64 (3): 1038-1044.

5. Fiatarone, M., E. O'Neill, N. Ryan et al. 1994. Exercise training and nutritional supplementation for physical frailty in very elderly people. *The New England Journal of Medicine* 330 (25): 1169-1175.

6. Faigenbaum, A., L. Zaichkowsky, W. Westcott et al. 1993. The effects of a twice-a-week strength training program on children. *Pediatric Exercise Science* 5: 339-346.

7. Westcott, W. 1994. Studies show significant gains in young muscles. *Nautilus* 3: 2, 6-7.

8. ———. 1995. Women vs. men: Are women really the weaker sex? *Nautilus* 4 (4): 3-5.

9. Sharkey, B.J. 1990. *Physiology of fitness.* 3d Ed. Champaign, IL: Human Kinetics.

10. Wilmore, J.H., and D.L. Costill. 1994. *Physiology of sport and exercise.* Champaign, IL: Human Kinetics.

11. Halloszy, J.O. 1967. Biomechanical adaptations in muscle: Effects of exercise on mitochondrial oxygen uptake and respiratory enzyme activity in skeletal muscle. *Journal of Biological Chemistry* 242: 2278-2282.

12. *University of California at Berkeley Wellness Letter.* 1995. Young at 70. 11 (May): 2-3.

Chapter 2

1. Westcott, W. 1995. *Strength fitness: Physiological principles and training techniques.* 4th Ed. Dubuque, IA: Brown and Benchmark.

2. Faigenbaum, A., L. Zaichkowsky, W. Westcott et al. 1992. Effects of twice per week strength training program on children. Paper presented at the annual meeting of the New England Chapter of American College of Sports Medicine, 12 November, at Boxborough, Massachusetts.

3. Westcott, W. 1995. Keeping fit. *Nautilus* 4 (2): 5-7.

4. Darden, E. 1987. *The Nautilus diet.* Boston: Little, Brown & Company.

5. Sheridan, S., T. Dohmeier, and J. Cleland. 1995. Effect of biometrics on body composition, strength, and blood lipid changes in middle age women. *Medicine and Science in Sports and Exercise* 27 (5): S140 Supplement.

6. Westcott, W. 1993. Weight gain and weight loss. *Nautilus* 3 (1): 8-9.

7. Evans, W., I. Rosenberg. 1992. *Biomarkers*. New York: Simon & Schuster.

8. Keyes, A., H.L. Taylor, and F. Grande. 1973. Basal metabolism and age of adult man. *Metabolism* 22: 579-587.

9. Melby, C., C. Scholl, G. Edwards et al. 1993. Effect of acute resistance exercise on postexercise energy expenditure and resting metabolic rate. *Journal of Applied Physiology* 75 (4): 1847-1853.

10. Campbell, W., M. Crim, V. Young, and W. Evans. 1994. Increased energy requirements and changes in body composition with resistance training in older adults. *American Journal of Clinical Nutrition* 60: 167-175.

11. Risch, S., N. Nowell, M. Pollock et al. 1993. Lumbar strengthening in chronic low back pain patients. *Spine* 18: 232-238.

12. Menkes, A., S. Mazel, A. Redmond et al. 1993. Strength training increases regional bone mineral density and bone remodeling in middle-aged and older men. *Journal of Applied Physiology* 74: 2478-2484.

13. Hurley, B. 1994. Does strength training improve health status? *Strength and Conditioning Journal* 16: 7-13.

14. Koffler, K., A. Menkes, A. Redmond et al. 1992. Strength training accelerates gastrointestinal transit in middle-aged and older men. *Medicine and Science in Sports and Exercise* 24: 415-419.

15. Stone, M., D. Blessing, R. Byrd et al. 1982. Physiological effects of a short term resistive training program on middle-aged untrained men. *National Strength and Conditioning Association Journal* 4: 16-20.

16. Hurley, B., J. Hagberg, A. Goldberg et al. 1988. Resistance training can reduce coronary risk factors without altering $\dot{V}O_2$max or percent body fat. *Medicine and Science in Sports and Exercise* 20: 150-154.

17. *Tufts University Diet and Nutrition Letter*. 1994. Never too late to build up your muscle. 12 (September): 6-7.

18. Harris, K. and R. Holly. 1987. Physiological response to circuit weight training in borderline hypertensive subjects. *Medicine and Science in Sports and Exercise* 19: 246-252.

19. Westcott, W. 1993. Strength training and blood pressure response. *Nautilus* 2 (4): 8-9.

Chapter 3

1. Braith, R., J. Graves, M. Pollock et al. 1989. Comparison of two versus three days per week of variable resistance training during 10 and 18 week programs. *International Journal of Sports Medicine* 10: 450-454.

2. Westcott, W. 1995. *Strength fitness: Physiological principles and training techniques*. 4th Ed. Dubuque, IA: Brown and Benchmark.

3. ———. 1995. Keeping fit. *Nautilus* 4 (2): 5-7.

4. American College of Sports Medicine. 1990. The recommended quantity and quality of exercise for developing and maintaining cardiorespiratory and muscular fitness in healthy adults. *Medicine and Science in Sports and Exercise* 22: 265-274.

5. Westcott, W., K. Greenberger, and D. Milius. 1989. Strength training research: Sets and repetitions. *Scholastic Coach* 58: 98-100.

6. Starkey, D., M. Welsch, M. Pollock et al. 1994. Equivalent improvement in

strength following high intensity, low and high volume training. Paper presented at the annual meeting of the American College of Sports Medicine, 2 June, at Indianapolis, Indiana.

7. Westcott, W. 1993. How many repetitions? *Nautilus* 2 (3): 6-7.

8. ———. 1994. Exercise speed and strength development. *American Fitness Quarterly* 13 (3): 20-21.

9. Jones, A., M. Pollock, J. Graves et al. 1988. *Safe, specific testing and rehabilitative exercise for the muscles of the lumbar spine.* Santa Barbara, CA: Sequoia Communications.

10. Risch, S., N. Nowell, M. Pollock et al. 1993. Lumbar strengthening in chronic low back pain patients. *Spine* 18: 232-238.

11. Westcott, W. 1986. Integration of strength, endurance, and skill training. *Scholastic Coach* 55: 74.

12. ———. 1994. High intensity strength training. *Nautilus* 4 (1): 5-8.

Chapter 7

1. *Harvard Heart Letter.* 1995. Data debunk myths about heart disease. 5 (June): 1-3.

2. Powell, K.E., P.D. Thompson, C.J. Caspersen et al. 1987. Physical activity and the incidence of coronary heart disease. *Annual Reviews in Public Health* 8: 253-287.

3. Caspersen, C.J. 1987. Physical inactivity and coronary heart disease. *The Physician and Sportsmedicine* 15: 43-44.

4. Peters, R.K., L.D. Cady, Jr., D.P. Bischoff et al. 1983. Physical fitness and subsequent myocardial infarction in healthy workers. *JAMA* 249: 3052-3056.

5. Blair, S.N., H.W. Kohl, III, D.G. Paffenbarger, Jr. et al. 1989. Physical fitness and all-cause mortality: A prospective study of healthy men and women. *JAMA* 262: 2395-2401.

6. American College of Sports Medicine. 1990. The recommended quantity and quality of exercise for developing and maintaining cardiorespiratory and muscular fitness in healthy adults. *Medicine and Science in Sports and Exercise* 22: 265-274.

7. Fox, S.M., J.P. Naughton, and P.A. Gorman. 1972. Physical activity and cardiovascular health. *Modern Concepts of Cardiovascular Health* 41: 20.

8. Harris, K.A., and R.G. Holly. 1987. Physiological response to circuit weight training in borderline hypertensive subjects. *Medicine and Science in Sports and Exercise* 19: 246-252.

9. Westcott, W. 1993. Strength training and blood pressure response. *Nautilus* 2 (Fall): 8-9.

10. Seals, D.R., and J.M. Hagberg. 1984. The effect of exercise training on human hypertension: A review. *Medicine and Science in Sports and Exercise* 16: 207-215.

11. Goldberg, L., and D.L. Elliot. 1985. The effect of physical activity on lipid and lipoprotein levels. *Medical Clinics of North America* 69: 41-55.

12. Pomerleau, O., H. Scherzer, N. Grunberg et al. 1987. The effects of acute exercise on subsequent cigarette smoking. *Journal of Behavioral Medicine* 10: 117-127.

13. *Tufts University Diet and Nutrition Letter.* 1994. To diet or not? The experts battle it out. 12 (October): 3-6.

14. Zuti, W.B., and L. Golding. 1976. Comparing diet and exercise as weight reduction tools. *The Physician and Sportsmedicine* 4: 59-62.

15. Rippe, J.M. 1992. *The exercise exchange program.* New York: Simon & Schuster.

16. Westcott, W. 1993. Weight gain and weight loss. *Nautilus* 3 (Winter): 8-9.

17. Wilmore, J.H., and D.L. Costill. 1994. *Physiology of sport and exercise.* Champaign, IL: Human Kinetics.

18. Sharkey, B.J. 1990. *Physiology of fitness.* 3d Ed. Champaign, IL: Human Kinetics.

Chapter 8

1. American College of Sports Medicine. 1990. The recommended quantity and quality of exercise for developing and maintaining cardiorespiratory and muscular fitness in healthy adults. *Medicine and Science in Sports and Exercise* 22: 265-274.

2. Westcott, W. 1995. Research: The skate machine. *American Fitness Quarterly* 15 (April): 37-39.

3. Pollock, M.L., L.R. Gettman, M.D. Milesis et al. 1977. Effects of frequency and duration of training on attrition and incidence of injury. *Medicine and Science in Sports* 9: 31-36.

4. Porcari, J.P. 1994. Fat-burning exercise: Fit or farce. *Fitness Management* 10: 40-41.

Chapter 9

1. Westcott, W. 1991. Comparison of upright and recumbent cycling exercise. *American Fitness Quarterly* 10 (October): 36-38.

2. ———. 1995. From the world of research: The skate machine. *American Fitness Quarterly* 13: 20-21.

Chapter 12

1. Westcott, W. 1986. Integration of strength, endurance and skill training. *Scholastic Coach* 55 (May-June): 74.

2. ———. 1995. *Strength fitness: Physiological principles and training techniques.* 4th Ed. Dubuque, IA: Brown and Benchmark.

3. Hennessy, L., and A. Watson. 1994. The interference effects of training for strength and endurance simultaneously. *Journal of Strength and Conditioning Research* 81: 12-19.

4. McCarthy, J., J. Agre, B. Graf et al. 1995. Compatibility of adaptive responses with combining strength and endurance training. *Medicine and Science in Sports and Exercise* 273: 429-436.

5. Westcott, W. 1987. *Building strength at the YMCA.* Champaign, IL: Human Kinetics.

Chapter 13

1. Westcott, W. 1995. High-intensity strength training. *IDEA Personal Trainer* 6: 7, 9.

Appendix A

1. Zimmer, J. 1995. Our 3rd annual health club hot list. *Fitness Magazine*, September, 48-50.

Index

About Nautilus International

In 1970 Arthur Jones developed and sold the first Nautilus exercise machine designed to strengthen the torso muscles, releasing a revolution in health and fitness. This was the first strength building machine on the market to use eccentric cams to provide variable, balanced resistance against the full range of motion.

The design of Nautilus equipment has evolved over the past quarter century as researchers have learned more about all of the requirements for strength building exercise equipment. These requirements, which only the Nautilus equipment line comprehensively satisfies, include rotary resistance, direct resistance, variable resistance, balanced resistance, positive work, negative work, stretching, prestretching, resistance in the full-contracted position, and unrestricted speed of movement. In addition to strength building exercise machines, Nautilus International manufactures a range of machines designed to increase cardiovascular fitness. These machines include fully recumbent stationary bicycles, stairclimbers, treadmills, and the unique Nautilus Skate Machine. With the help of respected researchers like Dr. Wayne Westcott, Nautilus International continues to improve its product line.

The versatility of use and the quality of results that the Nautilus fitness system produces have led to many professional sports teams including Nautilus equipment in their athletes' physical strength and conditioning programs. It also has created tremendous interest and good will among the millions of nonathletes around the world. Nautilus equipment is available in schools, rehabilitation centers, hospitals, hotels, corporate buildings, clinics, clubs, or homes.

To get the most from your workout, it is important to use the Nautilus equipment correctly. Nautilus International trains its customers to properly use and maintain the equipment to safely maximize results. It also provides many other complementary information sources, seminars, textbooks, and training manuals, such as *Building Strength and Stamina: New Nautilus Training for Total Fitness*.

With more than 30 years in strength training as an athlete, coach, teacher, professor, researcher, writer, and speaker, **Wayne Westcott,** PhD, is recognized as a foremost authority on fitness.

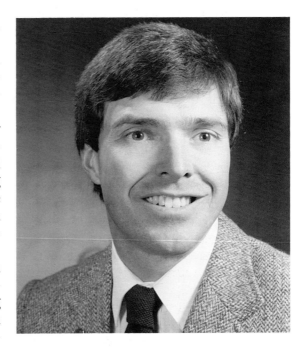

Westcott is fitness research director at the South Shore YMCA in Massachusetts, where he developed a model strength-fitness facility and training program rated the "Best Buy in the United States" by *Fitness Magazine* in 1995. This model is used as a prototype for designing fitness programs.

Westcott has served as a strength training consultant for numerous organizations and programs, including Nautilus, the President's Council on Physical Fitness and Sports, the International Association of Fitness Professionals (IDEA), the American Council on Exercise, the YMCA of the USA, the National Youth Sports Safety Foundation, and many others.

He was awarded the IDEA Lifetime Achievement Award in 1993 and was honored with a Healthy American Fitness Leader Award in 1995.

Westcott is highly sought after as a speaker and writer. He delivered the keynote address for the annual IDEA conference in 1995, and he lectures internationally on his research. He has written several books on strength training, including *Strength Fitness: Physiological Principles and Training Techniques*, a text physical education and exercise science majors have used for more than 15 years.

Since 1986 Westcott has written a weekly fitness column for one of the largest Boston area newspapers, the *Patriot Ledger.* The strength training advisor and fitness columnist for *Prevention* magazine, he also has served on the editorial boards of *Prevention, Shape, Men's Health, Fitness, Club Industry, American Fitness Quarterly,* and *Nautilus.*

Wescott lives in Abington, Massachusetts, with his wife, Claudia. He enjoys strength training, running, cycling, gardening, and volunteer work.

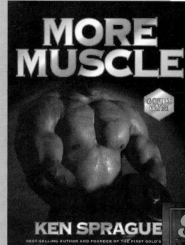
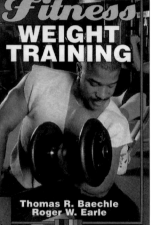
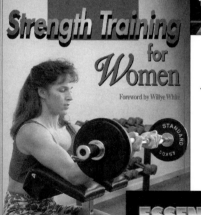
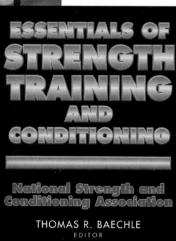